ADDICTED
HEALERS

ADDICTED HEALERS

*5 Key Signs Your Healthcare Professional
May Be Drug Impaired*

Ethan O. Bryson, MD

New Horizon Press
Far Hills, NJ

Requests for permission should be addressed to:
New Horizon Press
P.O. Box 669
Far Hills, NJ 07931

Ethan O. Bryson, MD
Addicted Healers:
5 Key Signs Your Healthcare Professional May Be Drug Impaired

Cover design: Bob Aulicino
Interior design: Scribe Inc.

Library of Congress Control Number: 2012932036

ISBN 13: 978-0-88282-392-8
New Horizon Press

Manufactured in the U.S.A.

16   15   14   13   12   1   2   3   4   5

For my wife Amity, our son Brady and our mom Linda.

Your love and support not only makes my work possible but also makes it worthwhile.

AUTHOR'S NOTE

This book is based on the author's research, personal experience, interviews and real life experiences. In order to protect privacy, names have been changed and identifying characteristics have been altered except for some contributing experts.

For purposes of simplifying usage, the pronouns his/her and s/he are sometimes used interchangeably. The information contained herein is not meant to be a substitute for professional evaluation and therapy with mental health professionals.

CONTENTS

Contents

Part V
What Needs to Be Done

PREFACE

D r. Bernard's day began at 4:30 A.M. when his bedside alarm interrupted his fifth hour of sleep. Most nights he was able to get six, sometimes seven hours straight, provided his child wasn't ill or the dog didn't need to go out, but the previous night had been another late night at the hospital and he hadn't gotten home until after ten. It seemed that he barely had enough time to recover each night before he had to return to work. Things had been changing a lot in his practice lately—in everyone's practices, it seemed—and there were more and more of these long working days each year. On top of this, the insurance companies continued to cut their reimbursements for his services and Medicare no longer covered the costs of providing care to his patients. So it was in this context of reduced income and increased responsibility that Dr. Bernard wondered how he was going to come up with enough money to make his mortgage payment, cover the costs of his son's special education and still be able to pay all of his monthly bills.

By 6:00 A.M., after a shower and two cups of coffee during the drive into the city, Dr. Bernard had reached the hospital, had changed into scrubs and was examining the day's schedule of cases. As the clinical coordinator, he was the attending anesthesiologist responsible for maintaining the flow of one of the busiest hospital-based operating facilities in the city. His group provided coverage for over fifty different operating rooms within the main hospital as well as several off-site locations, including the radiology department, where MRIs (magnetic resonance imaging) and CAT scans (computed axial tomography) were performed, the special procedures suites, where interventional radiologists coiled cerebral aneurysms and cardiologists performed catheterizations, and the labor floor, which consisted of fifteen labor and delivery rooms and three special operating rooms devoted entirely to pregnant patients.

Raul Sanchez had not been able to sleep at all. The pain in his gut kept getting worse and he had to get out of bed to go to the bathroom every hour or so. He tried to convince himself that it was the Chinese take-out food he and his wife had for dinner that night that had done this to him, but he had been sick with food poisoning before and this felt different. He couldn't identify exactly how it was different, because the pain was distracting him enough so that he couldn't really think straight, but he had a feeling of impending doom, like something terrible was about to happen. At 5:20 A.M., the world seemed to grow dim briefly and then he fell backwards into unconsciousness. Irma, who up until then had been sleeping soundly despite her husband's constant movement in and out of bed, awoke with a start. After forty-five years of marriage they shared a bond that ran deeper than most. Immediately she knew that something was not right. The light was on in the bathroom down the hall, so she could see well enough as she turned to look at her husband. He was completely still and looked almost gray. Irma shook Raul frantically but could not wake him up. In an instant she was out of bed and running into the kitchen, where their only telephone sat on the counter by the sink. Irma called 911. The operator dispatched an ambulance and then calmly told Irma what she needed to do for her husband. She ran back into the bedroom to check on him. Raul was not breathing; at least she didn't think he was, but how could she know? She checked his wrist but could not find a pulse either. The operator had said to breathe for him and then to push on his chest. Irma tried her best until the paramedics arrived.

By 5:35 A.M., Raul was on a stretcher in the back of an ambulance racing toward the hospital where Dr. Bernard practiced. Irma sat in the back of the rig and watched as one paramedic carefully placed a breathing tube in her husband while the other continued to press violently on his chest. A fireman was driving and, as he raced against the early morning traffic, the paramedics raced to save Raul's life. Within ten minutes the ambulance arrived at the hospital and before the paramedics could carry Raul out of the rig, Dr. Wu, an emergency medicine physician, was examining him. Dr. Wu conducted an ultrasound examination which confirmed the diagnosis: Raul's aorta, the largest artery in the body that connects directly to the heart, had ruptured. He needed emergency surgery and he needed it fast if he was going to survive. Dr. Wu's resident physician alerted the surgical resident on call and prepared to transport Raul up to the operating suite.

The ambulatory and day-of-surgery admission patients had already begun to arrive and the holding area, where patients were interviewed prior to entering the operating rooms, was filling up. As Dr. Bernard was checking the overnight messages from the answering service to learn who had called out sick and what cases had been added to his already unreasonably full schedule, he heard an emergency call from one of the surgical services. A patient had arrived in the emergency room with a ruptured abdominal aortic aneurysm and was being rushed to the operating room in an effort to save his life. Dr. Bernard heard the transport elevator across from the control desk begin to move. It would reach the emergency department three floors below in less than a minute, at which point the critically ill and most likely unstable patient would be loaded into the elevator and begin the ascent back to the third floor. He figured this gave him a little over two minutes to prepare to receive this patient. Dr. Bernard quickly sent a page to the overnight anesthesia team that was still on call and should still be in the hospital before running to get the operating room ready.

The nursing coordinator had assigned this case to the room directly across from the elevator and, as Dr. Bernard pushed open the doors and adjusted the mask on his face, he noted with a smile that the surgical technician and circulating nurse were quickly setting out all the sterile equipment that would be needed. The anesthesia equipment technician, a seasoned operating room veteran himself, was quickly running the anesthesia machine through the preoperative check, ensuring the breathing circuit was intact and that the equipment was functioning properly. Dr. Bernard opened the top drawer of the anesthesia supply cart and removed the medications he would need to keep the patient alive while the surgeons worked to repair the torn major vessel: epinephrine, norepinephrine and vasopressin to maintain blood pressure; vecuronium to provide paralysis and allow the surgeons to operate; scopolamine to provide amnesia just in case the patient couldn't tolerate any anesthesia. As he drew these medications into syringes, he carefully labeled each with the name of the drug and the exact concentration. Since doses of most anesthetic agents are based on weight, Dr. Bernard would have to calculate quickly the appropriate amount of each drug to administer after the patient arrived.

Outside the operating room, the early morning quiet was broken by a soft ping announcing that the transport elevator had returned to the third floor. Dr. Bernard took a deep breath, held it and then exhaled. All hell was about to break loose. Five seconds later, the double doors to the operating room swung inward as the transport stretcher pushed them out of the way. Raul lay motionless on the wheeled gurney. Dr. Bernard noted that a breathing tube had already been placed. That was good; one less thing to worry about. Two large-bore intravenous lines had been attached, probably by the paramedics in the field. Blood was rapidly flowing through one and a balanced salt solution through the other. Both the blood and the fluid were being administered under high pressure in an attempt to replace the blood that was ejected from the patient's torn aorta with every beat of his rapidly failing heart. Attached to the breathing tube was a self-inflating manual resuscitation bag. Every few seconds, one of the surgical residents squeezed the bag and delivered 100 percent oxygen under positive pressure to the patient's lungs. Another surgical resident straddled the patient on the stretcher performing cardiopulmonary resuscitation (CPR), compressing the patient's chest eighty to one hundred times per minute.

The team of nurses and doctors from the emergency department and surgical services worked well together. Even though some had never met and few had ever run a code together, everyone knew exactly what to do and there was little need to talk or ask questions. In one fluid movement, the transporter moved the gurney against the operating room table at just the right position so that when Raul was lifted onto the table he would not have to be readjusted. As Dr. Bernard began to apply his monitors—electrocardiogram stickers to monitor the electrical activity of the heart, pulse oximeter to measure the oxygen saturation and blood pressure cuff—the emergency department nurse removed the monitors that had to be returned to the emergency room with the transport monitor. Up until this moment, the senior surgical resident had been directing the management of the patient, but now that Raul was in his operating room, Dr. Bernard was in charge of running the code. Recognizing this transfer of authority, the resident then gave Dr. Bernard a brief history of what they knew and what they expected to find, before heading out of the room to scrub.

The surgical resident who had been managing the airway handed the bag to Dr. Bernard, who attached the breathing tube to the anesthesia machine, turned on the ventilator and directed the team to move the patient from the stretcher to the table. The resident performing CPR dropped to the opposite side of the table and grabbed the draw sheet below Raul. On Dr. Bernard's count, four people lifted Raul onto the operating room table in one synchronized motion and began to prepare for the initial surgical incision. Just then, the on call attending physician and one of the senior anesthesia residents burst through the doors and moved to where Dr. Bernard was working at the head of the bed. While the on call attending took report, preparing to assume responsibility for the case, the resident placed an arterial line in Raul's arm so they could monitor blood pressure on a beat-by-beat basis and a processed encephalogram probe on the patient's forehead to monitor his brain activity.

Dr. Bernard, the on call anesthesia team, the surgeons, the nurses and the operating room technicians all worked tirelessly for the next two hours and were eventually able to save Raul's life. His surgery began less than forty-five minutes after he initially collapsed, a considerable feat given the number of people and resources that needed to be coordinated in such a short period of time. If you think this was the exception rather than the rule, then you're wrong. Despite the incredible challenges associated with providing health-care in a system complicated by ever-increasing demands, diminishing resources and decreased compensation and respect, today's healthcare providers continue to perform to the highest of standards. But such performance depends upon every person functioning at the highest level and being able to maintain that performance for an extended period of time. In the pressured, hectic atmosphere of the operating room, even during a routine case, a single slip or moment of inattention has the potential to compromise people's lives and health. In this environment, healthcare workers do not have the luxury of worrying about their personal problems or even about their work-related problems during working hours. Their attention must be on the patient at all times. To look away for even a minute can have disastrous consequences.

Imagine that one of the healthcare workers in this emergency case was impaired due to drug abuse. Would things have turned out differently for Raul? Would Irma still be sitting by Raul's hospital bed as he recovered from his life-saving surgery or would she be planning for his funeral? As we will see, medical professionals in our healthcare system have the potential to harm patients, both through their actions and through inaction, even if they never have the opportunity to handle a patient.

From the moment the first call is made to emergency medical services until the patient leaves the hospital, one important reason the patient's life is potentially in danger is not from what you might think. Imagine that one of the paramedics who arrived on the scene to care for Raul was a drug addict. It is then possible that the paramedic's judgment could have been clouded by intoxication or withdrawal. Perhaps the emergency medicine physician at the base hospital ordered the administration of a controlled drug like morphine, but the paramedic pocketed the drug himself and gave the patient saline instead. Sound implausible? It has happened many times before. What if the paramedic had diverted the morphine intended for her previous patient and had self-administered the morphine moments before getting the call for Raul's case? What if she had shot up the morphine hours before and was feeling the effects of narcotic withdrawal? Any number of possible dangerous scenarios exists, but no matter how each plays out, the risk that this impaired paramedic could injure the patient increases substantially, and this is only in the pre-hospital setting.

Once the patient arrives at the hospital, the number of healthcare professionals on whom this patient's life depends increases dramatically. The doctors and nurses in the emergency department and on the surgical service must all work together, functioning at the highest level, if they are going to save a critically ill patient's life. Impairment in any one of these professionals has the potential to affect this team's efforts tremendously. Decreased vigilance, miscalculations, delayed reaction times and diversion of critical drugs all have the potential to harm a patient. When a healthcare professional is under the influence of drugs, the odds that these types of errors will happen are high.

What if Dr. Bernard was an addict, concerned more with obtaining medications to prevent withdrawal or perhaps having just self-administered these drugs? In this situation, the slightest delay in making critical decisions regarding the management of the patient had the potential for disaster. What if he had not thought to call for assistance and was unable to manage this patient by himself? What if he had mislabeled the syringes containing the emergency medications and given Raul the wrong drug? What if he had gone to get high on drugs instead of to the control desk and was unavailable when the patient arrived in the operating room?

While some of the more dramatic stories of addicted healthcare professionals are those that involve addicted physicians and nurses whose impairment and mismanagement directly affects seriously ill patients, every impaired healthcare professional has the potential to cause harm. Does the radiologist on call get a free pass or could his drug use potentially cause harm to a patient? What if the radiologist, expecting a slow night with little responsibility, was drinking or using drugs in the warm shadows of the radiology department's reading room? What if, in this impaired state, the radiologist misreads the critical imaging test and does not diagnose a potentially life-threatening condition? What about the pharmacist? Even the pharmacist, far removed from direct patient contact, has the potential to make critical errors that can result in injury or death and thus cannot lower his or her attentiveness.

The potential for addiction among healthcare professionals represents a significant source of morbidity and mortality, both for the affected individuals and for the patients for whom they care. According to the United States Department of Health and Human Services, Substance Abuse and Mental Health Services Administration, rates of illicit drug use by healthcare professionals within the past year ranged from 8 percent to 20 percent depending on the type of personnel within the healthcare industry, with physicians, dentists and optometrists reporting use at the higher end of the range and therapists and technologists at the lower end.[1] At any given time, roughly 3 to 5 percent of this population is using illicit drugs while they are caring for patients. Healthcare professionals abuse alcohol and drugs at rates similar to the general population from which they come, but their dependence on prescription medications is higher.[2] It seems that individuals with access to prescription medications and a desire to get high choose these drugs over marijuana, cocaine, heroin or other street drugs.[3]

There is this myth in our society that the people who choose to become doctors, nurses and other healthcare workers are somehow different from everyone else. We hold these professionals to a much higher standard, because the stakes are so high and because we may not understand much of what they do; the trust implicit in this unbalanced relationship requires it. These individuals are entrusted with the care of the most vulnerable members of our society and regularly perform important work in highly safety-sensitive positions. Errors in diagnosis or treatment made by impaired healthcare professionals have implications which affect the health and well-being of all of us. Like workers in the aviation industry or military who must perform at a very high level or risk significant injury to large numbers of dependents, healthcare professionals do not have the luxury of reduced vigilance.

Throughout history, some healthcare professionals partook of their own medications, frequently to the point of severe impairment. Although many great medical breakthroughs were made because the physician scientists on the front lines of medicine were willing to experiment with new therapies, often on themselves, society no longer can accept this sort of experimentation and must curtail drug-impaired behavior among healthcare providers. When a healthcare professional is found to be impaired, we need more safeguards in place to move the addicted individual into treatment and out of the clinical arena.

PART I

THE SCOPE OF
THE EPIDEMIC

CHAPTER 1

Harm Caused by Addicted Healthcare Professionals

Television dramas like *Nurse Jackie* and *House*, both fictional accounts of addicted yet functioning healthcare professionals, present a side of healthcare that most people don't think of as real. Despite the premise that these shows are fictional, doctors, nurses, pharmacists, dentists, respiratory therapists, paramedics or anyone with access to highly addictive medications have the potential to abuse them. The very real death of pop-culture icon Michael Jackson and the conviction of his personal physician, Dr. Conrad Murray, for involuntary manslaughter dramatically illustrate the power these drugs have; even the slightest miscalculation has the potential to kill. Although Dr. Murray's actions were malpractice, he was not found to be impaired due to drug use himself. Yet the unfortunate result of his actions was the death of a publicly acclaimed and admired figure. When the healthcare professionals trusted with protecting our health and safety become addicted to powerful and dangerous drugs, the results can be devastating. Unfortunately, addiction to drugs is not an isolated incident or a rare event. Every day patients are put at risk by the very people with whom they trust their lives and their health.

Obstetrician and Speed Freak

As physician reimbursement continues to drop and doctors are required to see more and more patients each day, patients have become accustomed to longer waiting times and shorter visits. But sometimes it's not a need to ramp up productivity to cover costs that underlies these speedy patient encounters.

Amy, a thirty-two-year-old woman in her first trimester of pregnancy, developed some cramping and spotting and visited her obstetrician for evaluation. Amy's first pregnancy had been uncomplicated and she really liked Dr. Reese, the obstetrician who delivered her first baby, so when she found out she was pregnant again she returned to his care. "This was my second pregnancy, so it's not like I didn't know what was normal and what wasn't," Amy conveyed. "I went to see Dr. Reese because something wasn't right." In the two years since her first delivery the practice had grown considerably and Dr. Reese had taken on a second physician to handle the increased volume. When Amy came in for her evaluation, it was this second physician, Dr. Schwartz, who took care of her.

As Dr. Schwartz entered the exam room where Amy lay waiting for his arrival, he saw everything in exquisite detail. In an instant he noted an awkward curve in the window curtains and made a mental note to have them sent out to be re-stitched. Before he had crossed the room he had identified a chipped tile that should be replaced, a dust ball under the exam table that suggested the evening cleaning crew was somewhat less than thorough and several clear glass jars of medical supplies that needed to be refilled.

Dr. Schwarz quickly grabbed the probe, abruptly pulled up Amy's gown and sprayed a glob of jelly on her abdomen. It was as if his brain was moving faster than his body could. Lists of things to do, plans for the afternoon and later that evening and into the remainder of the year ran through his mind while he performed the routine ultrasound examination. He quickly found the fetal heartbeat and pronounced the pregnancy to be in good order. He was gone in an instant and Amy lay on the table, not quite sure what had just happened. "He seemed harried and stressed, but I thought that this was just what the practice was like now. There were so many people in the waiting room I just figured he didn't have the time to waste on small talk. He said everything looked good so I thought the cramping and spotting was okay and thought nothing more of it. He said that I should make an appointment to come back in three months."

Dr. Schwartz spent less than two minutes in the room with Amy before quickly returning to his office. Once the door was securely locked, he strode across the room to his desk, sat in his large leather-backed swivel chair and pulled open the lower drawer on the right-hand side. After moving aside a stack of charts, Dr. Schwartz removed an ornately engraved wooden box a patient had brought him from somewhere in South America. He placed the box on the desk in front of him, beginning what had become a ritual he performed several times a day. He removed the lid by sliding it out of the tight grooves that kept it secure when it was in place and moved it to the side, focusing now on the contents of the box. Inside the wooden box was a metal box with a metal clasp, a mirror, a straw and a razor blade. Dr. Schwartz removed the four items one by one and placed them on the desk in front of him. Then he moved the wooden box to the side and opened the clasp on the metal box. A white powder filled the inside of the second box and he used the razor blade to scoop out a portion onto the mirror. Confident that he had removed enough of the powder, he closed the metal box and, after securing the clasp, placed it back into the wooden box. A smile crept across his face as he used the razor blade to form a thin line of the powdered methamphetamine. Leaning over the mirror, he caught a glimpse of himself just before inhaling. He looked amazing, so powerful and confident. He felt as though he could do anything. Dr. Schwartz wiped what little powder remained on the mirror into the wooden box and then placed the mirror, straw and razor blade inside. Reattaching the lid on the wooden box, he returned it to its proper place under the stack of patient charts in his desk drawer, unlocked the door and moved quickly down the hallway to see the next patient.

Unfortunately, Amy did not get better. One week after Dr. Schwartz had pronounced her pregnancy to be in good order, Amy collapsed at the dinner table. Fearing for her life, her husband called an ambulance and Amy was rushed to the emergency room with symptoms of a ruptured ectopic pregnancy. In this case, the embryo had become implanted in the fallopian tube and not in the uterus as it should have. As the embryo continued to grow it became too large for the narrow tube in which it was growing, resulting in the cramping and spotting that had prompted Amy's first visit to her obstetrician. The ultrasound Dr. Schwartz performed should have found the ectopic pregnancy. He should have known that this degree of cramping and spotting during the first trimester was unusual and been more careful to identify a cause. In this case, he was more concerned with getting back to his office where he could continue to use methamphetamine and his diagnostic error resulted in a catastrophe for Amy. "As soon as I got to the emergency room they did another ultrasound and I was brought upstairs immediately for emergency surgery. I thank God that Dr. Schwartz was not on call that night. I may have died."

Amy survived the operation, but not without significant cost. Because Dr. Schwartz had failed to diagnose the ectopic pregnancy at the initial presentation and treat the problem in a timely fashion, an emergency hysterectomy had to be performed. As a result of this physician's diagnostic error, directly related to his abuse of methamphetamine, Amy lost not only this pregnancy, but also the ability to have children in the future. "My husband and I were devastated. We had planned to have a large family. I'm thankful that we have one child and that I'm alive, but when I think back on what happened I still get angry. This was a preventable thing; it didn't have to happen." Amy and her husband sued Dr. Schwartz and his malpractice insurance carrier settled the case without going to trial. "The important thing, though, is that this guy is not practicing anymore. They won't tell me where he is or what he is doing, but according to the state medical board he turned in his license." Amy's story is just one of many examples of the harm which can result from the abuse of drugs or alcohol by a healthcare professional.

Pharmacist and Pill Thief

When we think of someone being injured by an impaired healthcare professional, what comes to mind is usually that the doctor or the nurse was high on drugs and not able to provide the patient the care we expect, but even those professionals peripherally involved in patient care have the potential to cause great harm.

Kathy, a twenty-five-year-old widow, lost her husband, the father of her two young children, as the direct result of an error propagated by an impaired pharmacist. "Doug was carrying the patio furniture in off the back porch for the winter and he must have hurt a muscle in his back. He's never had anything like that happen before, so when it didn't get better I told him he should see his doctor. The doc said it wasn't anything serious but gave him a prescription for pain medication." Kathy took Doug's prescription to a pharmacy close to the doctor's office to be filled. "We usually go to the pharmacy near our home," she explained, "but Doug was in a lot of pain, so I wanted him to be able to take something for the ride home." Doug's prescription was filled by Mr. Patel, the pharmacist at this new pharmacy, who inadvertently dispensed pills ten times the dose of the narcotic medication Doug's doctor had prescribed. Kathy revealed, "Doug took two of the pills in the car as soon as I got the prescription filled. By the time we got home he was very groggy, so I helped him upstairs to our bed so he could rest. He never woke up."

An investigation revealed that the prescription had been written correctly but that Mr. Patel had misread the doctor's instructions and dispensed what amounted to a lethal dose of medication for someone with no tolerance for narcotics. When interviewed, Mr. Patel reported that Kathy had been "very demanding" and "impatient" and that he felt hurried and just "wanted her to go away." But the results of a for-cause urine screening indicated that Mr. Patel had been abusing the same narcotic medication. The investigation determined that the error resulted directly from Mr. Patel's misuse of prescription narcotic medications which he had been diverting from the pharmacy stock. "My husband is dead and this was completely preventable. What am I supposed to do now?" Kathy has been left to raise her two young children. Funds from the legal settlement have been placed in trusts for each of her children and she has enough money to support herself as a result of the lawsuit, but no amount of money can replace the father of these children. "They are never going to know their daddy anymore; you can't put a price on that. It all seems so random and meaningless."

As this example shows, medical errors can occur at any link along the chain of patient care and sometimes the results of these errors are deadly. Protocols designed to prevent this kind of error would have had Mr. Patel verify the prescription with the prescribing physician if the dose seemed too high, but it is unclear whether he simply grabbed the wrong strength pills from pharmacy stock or misread the prescription and didn't bother to check with the physician. In either case, the error was likely made because Mr. Patel was affected by the narcotic medication he was using and was not alert.

Fentanyl Abusing Anesthesia Resident

Medication errors can happen when the patient is administered the wrong medication, the wrong dose of the right medication, the right medication at the wrong time or no medication at all. Since humans are not infallible, safeguards have been put in place to prevent patient harm resulting from human error. Think of these safeguards that have been put in place, such as reading the patient's nametag prior to administering any medication, checking the vial of medication to ensure it is the correct drug and verifying the dose with the pharmacy, as slices of Swiss cheese. These Swiss cheese slices represent the tasks that must be accomplished prior to medication administration. Each safeguard is designed to prevent an error, but just as Swiss cheese has holes, these safety checks are not perfect barriers by themselves. When multiple slices are piled together, however, the odds are that an error that passes through a hole in one slice will be blocked by the next slice. Unfortunately, sometimes the Swiss cheese slices line up just so and it is up to healthcare professionals to recognize and stop errors before they reach the patients. When the person in charge is an addicted healthcare professional, it's only a matter of time before someone gets hurt or worse.

Brigit, a morbidly obese forty-five-year-old woman, was given the wrong medication before her weight loss surgery. "I was brought into the operating room by the anesthesia resident, Dr. Brown, a very nice young man who seemed very concerned about my comfort and well-being," Brigit explained. "He put the monitors on and started an intravenous line, at which point another, older man came in and introduced himself as Dr. Jeffery. He said he was the attending anesthesiologist and asked if I had any questions. I said no and they placed a mask over my face and asked me to take several deep breaths. I thought I would be going to sleep, but suddenly I got the worst headache I have ever had. It was as if my head was going to explode." As soon as Brigit reported her symptoms, the anesthetic induction was aborted and the doctors began to treat her symptoms and try to figure out what had gone wrong. "Things began to get very tense. It was as if they knew something bad was happening. They kept telling me everything was going to be alright, but I really didn't believe them. They started poking my wrist to put in more monitoring lines and they were giving me medications through the intravenous and eventually I began to feel better, but they decided it would be better not to do the surgery on that day."

Brigit had received several standard medications through the intravenous line as part of the pre-induction phase of anesthesia. One of the medications, metoclopramide, is given to reduce the chance that anything that might be in a patient's stomach will come up into the patient's mouth and subsequently enter the lungs during the operation, an event called aspiration which often has disastrous consequences and can result in death. Unfortunately, in Brigit's case the doctors discovered that an error commonly referred to as a "syringe swap" had occurred and Brigit had not received metoclopramide. Instead, Dr. Brown had drawn up another medication, phenylephrine, from a vial that looked very similar to the metoclopramide vial, and administered that instead. Phenylephrine is a medication that is commonly used to support a patient's blood pressure during anesthesia, but it must first be diluted. Not only had Brigit received the wrong medication, but also she had received one hundred times the standard dose. The result was a hypertensive crisis during which her blood pressure skyrocketed. "At first my surgeon told me that I had had an allergic reaction to one of the drugs that the anesthesia team had given me, but later, in the recovery room, Dr. Brown came to me and explained what had really happened. He seemed so nervous and scared; I thought he was going to cry. Even though his error had almost killed me, I felt bad for him."

Thankfully, Brigit suffered no permanent harm from this incident and returned to have her surgery successfully completed the following week. A root cause analysis determined that the error was the end result of a policy that allowed a potentially dangerous medication to remain in its undiluted form adjacent to other "look-alike" medications in the anesthesia cart, but a for-cause urine screening revealed that Dr. Brown had been abusing fentanyl and he was subsequently referred for treatment.

In Brigit's story, it is uncertain what role the substance abuse by the resident played in the resulting patient harm. The lack of vigilance on the part of the resident, who drew up the incorrect medication, contributed to the error. Had he been able to prevent the propagation, this event would have been classified as a "near-miss" had it been reported, rather than the sentinel event it turned out to be. But a problem existed. Unfortunately, the findings of the root cause analysis, which determined that an unsafe condition existed, were overshadowed by the discovery that the resident had been abusing fentanyl and any motivation to change hospital policy or procedures was lost. Sadly, the unsafe conditions remained in place and, three years later, the same error was made, this time by an attending who was determined to be free of the influence of drug abuse. A second root cause analysis determined that the same unsafe conditions existed and again recommended a change in policy. Unfortunately, this was too late to prevent the death of the second patient, who fell victim to the same error.

Certified Registered Nurse Anesthetist and Junkie

At a different hospital in a different city, the same systems, put in place to prevent a medication error, were unable to save the life of one patient who suffered irreparable harm due to a syringe swap error made by a nurse anesthetist who had been abusing prescription medications.

William had been told by his orthopedic surgeon that the arthritis in his knees, the result of considerable trauma during his career as a semi-professional athlete, had reached the point where he needed a knee replacement. The operation was simple, one that the surgeon had performed many times before and typically required no more than a spinal anesthetic. A small needle placed in the back, through which local anesthesia is injected into the spinal canal, would provide enough anesthesia for the procedure. William could remain awake but not feel anything while his knee was being replaced.

On the day of the surgery, the assignment to provide anesthesia fell to Sarah, a certified registered nurse anesthesiologist (CRNA), who, unbeknownst to anyone, had been diverting and self-injecting narcotics. In this particular practice, the CRNA was not required to be supervised by a physician anesthesiologist and the attending surgeon typically took on that role, though his knowledge of anesthesia was considerably less than hers. Though physician anesthesiologists were available for consult should she require it, as a senior nurse anesthetist Sarah rarely sought their advice or assistance with basic cases such as this. When the spinal had been placed successfully, she turned her attention to trying to figure out how she could obtain the drugs she needed for herself. Sarah had been assigned to an ortho-pedic room for the day and because these cases were typically done with spinals or epidurals, even the large cases required very little nar-cotics. The way she normally obtained these drugs was to indicate on the medical chart that she had given them to her patients but then keep the narcotics for herself. In cases where the primary anesthetic was spinal, very little narcotics were required and Sarah knew she wouldn't be able to get enough of the drug. This worried her, because she was already feeling the effects of withdrawal.

Sarah was becoming physically ill. She was already beginning to feel cold. Sarah looked down and saw gooseflesh; the hairs on her arms were all erect. She knew the vague nausea and aching in her bones was just the beginning. Sarah had been through narcotic withdrawal before and she knew that if she didn't get more of the drugs she needed she wouldn't be able to make it through the day.

As Sarah tried to think of a way out of this situation, she heard the surgeon ask for two grams of cefazolin and she reached into the drawer of the anesthesia cart to draw up the antibiotic for injection. The drug existed in a powdered form and she reconstituted the agent with saline from a prefilled syringe as she had done several times a day for many years. The actions were unconscious and her body per-formed them without thought or consideration. As she popped off the cap to the ampule, she was distracted and did not notice that the color of the top was red and not the white that it should have been. As she drew the reconstituted liquid into the syringe she looked at the bottle but did not read the label. She did not notice that she had drawn up ten milligrams of vecuronium, a powerful paralytic agent, and not the cefazolin antibiotic she had intended to. Not paying attention to what she was doing, she tossed the now empty ampule in the waste container and injected the medication.

Vecuronium is not intended to be administered to a patient who is awake; it paralyzes the skeletal muscles and prevents the patient from being able to move, but it is not an anesthetic. Patients who receive this drug cannot breathe or move. If they have not also received anesthesia, they remain wide awake and fully aware of what is going on. Full muscle paralysis is required for many surgeries, but vecuronium is always administered after the patient has entered a state of general anesthesia and is unaware of what is going on.

This drug typically takes about three minutes to work fully, but in this case it is likely that William, who was already paralyzed from the waist down because of the spinal anesthesia, began to feel weak shortly after the unintended dose had been administered. As the vecuronium began to work, he probably noticed some difficulty breathing. Perhaps he tried to voice his concerns to Sarah but, being weak as he was, could not make a sound. It is impossible to know how he felt or what he thought in those minutes as he lay awake and paralyzed, unable to breathe. Being a healthy man with no other medical problems, it took a long time for the monitors to show signs of his deteriorating state. By the time the alarms that indicated William's oxygen saturation levels and heart rate were too low caught Sarah's attention, it was too late.

William suffered a hypoxic cardiac arrest, meaning his heart was starved for oxygen and eventually stopped working properly. Sarah and her backup team eventually successfully resuscitated William, but not before his brain was severely damaged from the extended period of time without oxygen. He did not survive.

Such an error may or may not have been preventable, but at the very least it should have been noticed long before the patient deteriorated to the point where he suffered irreparable brain damage. This error claimed Sarah's life too. Unable to live with the consequences of her actions and the knowledge of the horrific way in which William died, awake and suffocating, unable to breathe, Sarah later administered the same drug to herself but followed it with an induction dose of propofol. She rapidly entered a state of general anesthesia from which she never woke up.

While dramatic, these examples of how addicted healthcare professionals can directly impact patients' health and safety are not works of fiction. Despite the multitude of safeguards that have been put in place to prevent patient harm from occurring, thousands of patients are injured each year as a direct result of medical errors. The Committee on Quality of Health Care in America and Institute of Medicine report titled *To Err Is Human: Building a Safer Health System* suggests that unintentional patient harm due to medical errors may be responsible for the death of at least 44,000 people and perhaps as many as 98,000 people each year.[1] A similar report published in the New England Journal of Medicine in 2010 claims that as much as 25 percent of patients may be harmed in some way during their inpatient hospitalization, suggesting that little progress has been made despite a call to reduce the number of preventable errors and decrease patient harm.[2] Errors, such as preventable adverse drug events, improper transfusions, surgical injuries, wrong-site surgery, restraint-related injuries, falls, burns, pressure ulcers and mistaken patient identities, were cited as examples of the kinds of events which ultimately lead to death or serious injury. The majority of medical errors do not result from one person's actions. More commonly, errors are caused by faulty systems, processes and conditions that lead people to make mistakes or fail to prevent them. In some ways, healthcare practitioners are set up to fail, but these types of errors also result from the decreased vigilance that is the hallmark of addicted healthcare professionals. It is very likely that some of these errors are the direct result of illicit drug use.

When errors occur, they are the end result of a chain of events which allows the propagation of incorrect thoughts or actions. The severity of patient harm, if harm occurs, or risk of harm, if the error is prevented, depends on the links in the chain and the direction of the propagation. For example, unsafe conditions may be created by limited knowledge of how a potentially dangerous device, such as a carbon dioxide laser, functions or what safety precautions are necessary when the device is powered on. Perhaps the device is a newer model and the surgeon or surgical technician is not familiar with the new arrangements of the controls or the safety features. Having a representative from the manufacturer on site to explain the proper functioning of the device's controls as it is used can reduce the risk for patient harm and eliminate the unsafe conditions.

The existence of two or more medications with look-alike containers in the same stockroom can lead to the delivery of the wrong medication to the patient. In most situations, there are multiple steps during which safety checks are performed to ensure that medication errors do not occur. The physician who places the order must verify that the ordered medication is the correct concentration and that there are no contraindications, such as allergies or incompatibility with other medications the patient may be taking. These checks are often performed by a computer with prompts delivered to the prescribing physician in real time as the orders are entered. Once the order is received by the pharmacist, protocols are followed to ensure that the medication dispensed from hospital supplies is correct and that the container, infusion bag or syringe is labeled correctly.

Before the medication is administered to the patient, a final check is performed by the nurse to ensure that the medication is actually intended for this patient and not the patient in the next room or one with a similar name on a different floor. Along the chain of propagation, any link has the power to identify and stop the error, but when the chain is short or safety checks are bypassed, the end result can be disastrous. Each safety check provides the opportunity for someone to catch the error or, if they are not vigilant, to propagate it.

Diagnostic errors result from factors such as a delay in diagnosis, a failure to employ or properly interpret indicated tests or a failure to act on results of proper monitoring or tests. In the hurried and high-pressure environment in which healthcare is delivered today, it is not uncommon to encounter these types of errors. For the most part, they are minor deviations from the standard of care with little clinical consequence, but occasionally very real harm occurs and sometimes this is the end result of a series of errors propagated by an impaired healthcare professional. Treatment errors can occur during the performance of an operation, procedure or test. An avoidable delay in treatment, a delay in responding to an abnormal test or an error in the administration of the treatment, such as the wrong dose of a medication, can result in significant harm to the patient.

Treatment errors in the form of the administration of the incorrect concentration or dose of a medication are more common than they should be and sometimes result from the actions of impaired healthcare professionals. Given how commonly syringe swap errors occur, it is surprising that they are not reported more often, but perhaps this is because many swaps have little clinical consequence. Once a clear liquid drug is drawn into a syringe, the only thing distinguishing it from another clear liquid drug, at least to the naked eye, is the label placed on the syringe by the person who drew up the drug. Drugs are often obtained in bulk by the hospital pharmacy from different manufacturers depending on who has the best price. There is little consistency of packaging across drug companies and when it's time to reorder a particular drug, the packaging may have changed, so healthcare professionals who are putting the drugs in the syringes must remain vigilant. In reality, these types of errors probably occur more often than we know, probably because they frequently do not have any clinical consequences. But sometimes, as we have seen, a syringe swap can result in patient harm and this can have profound implications.

Preventive failures occur when an avoidable disease is not prevented. Errors that result in inadequate treatment, inadequate follow-up of treatment or failure to provide preventive treatment when indicated can result in significant patient harm. This can happen even if the correct diagnosis is made or when the indicated test is performed but no action is taken based on the results of the test or diagnosis. In the case of the methamphetamine abusing obstetrician we discussed earlier, the correct diagnosis was never made. What if the diagnosis had been made based on the proper exam but no action was taken based on those results? It is unlikely that this would happen in an emergency situation, although when drugs are involved even the unlikely is possible. Errors related to equipment failures, system failures or failures of communication can also result in significant patient harm and may result directly from an impaired member of the healthcare delivery team anywhere along the chain.

CHAPTER 2

A Problem More Common than You Think

Addicted healthcare professionals practice in a context of mass addiction. Prescription drug abuse represents a serious and growing public health problem, not only in the United States, but in most other parts of the world as well. People from all social strata are becoming addicted to these medications and the number of addicts is increasing at an alarming rate.[1] While lifetime use of heroin in the United States increased from 1.2 percent of the population in the year 2000 to 1.5 percent in 2005, the nonmedical use of prescription narcotics increased from 8.6 percent to 13.4 percent over the same five-year period.[2]

The increase in prescription drug abuse is a worldwide phenomenon. According to a 2006 report published by the International Narcotics Control Board, prescription drug abuse is increasing in most countries in Europe, Africa and South Asia as addicts move away from traditional illicitly produced drugs like cocaine and heroin and toward prescription medications like fentanyl and oxycodone.[3] Even as efforts aimed at repurposing the poppy fields in Afghanistan and managing coca production in Bolivia have reduced the supply of heroin and cocaine available on the world market, addicts are increasing their consumption of prescription drug alternatives.

This substantial increase in medication misuse is not an isolated trend and the problem appears to be getting worse. Highly addictive prescription narcotics are increasingly available from multiple sources, including friends and family members who have been legitimately prescribed these medications. Narcotics once reserved for those with terminal cancer are increasingly prescribed for chronic pain, leading to greater availability of these medications and presenting greater opportunity for misuse.[4]

The misuse of drugs with legitimate medical uses is called diversion. These drugs are prescribed for one use, often to treat pain, but they are subsequently diverted for another use: to get high. The rise of Internet pharmacies with questionable prescribing practices, offering prescriptions with minimal physician contact to anyone with a credit card, further exacerbates this problem. With such increased availability, today's addict no longer fits the classic stereotype of the down-and-out individual who is living on the outskirts of society. However, the last people we would expect to become addicted to these medications are the ones whom we charge with prescribing and administering them.

Traveling Physician in Search of Drugs

The risk that an impaired healthcare professional will harm a patient is not limited only to the direct contact that surgical and other hospital-based practices have. When these professionals are impaired, the number of prescriptions they write for highly addictive medications increases considerably. Ronald, a recent retiree who had moved to Florida from New Jersey, developed what he thought was indigestion one evening after a particularly heavy meal. Despite not having exercised regularly for the majority of his life, he thought that perhaps a short walk with his dog would settle his stomach. After a block he found he couldn't keep up. Short of breath and sweating profusely, he sat down on the curb and called his wife, who called an ambulance. Ronald was brought to the community hospital with symptoms suggesting he was having a heart attack. Overweight and with high cholesterol and high blood pressure, he was a setup for heart failure.

To the paramedics who brought him to the hospital the diagnosis was clear, but in the emergency room the physician was not so convinced. Dr. Thomas had recently moved back to Florida himself and was having trouble adjusting to the types of patients he was now seeing. Unlike the small community hospital in California where he had practiced for a decade, the people who came into this ER were much older and altogether sicker.

Dr. Thomas had left his practice in California rather abruptly when it became clear to him that the state medical board was investigating his prescribing practices. The board had become suspicious when a pharmacist reported that a number of prescriptions for narcotics written for different patients had been filled by what appeared to be the same person. Dr. Thomas had been writing prescriptions for his friends and himself using the names of patients who came into his emergency department. He figured that since the population was primarily migrant farm workers and homeless people with nowhere else to go for healthcare that it would be hard for anyone to figure out what he was doing. The prescriptions were not forged and the names were real people if anyone checked, but he hadn't counted on the pharmacist noticing who was actually filling them. By the time he realized that an investigation had been initiated, Thomas was too addicted to stop.

Strung out on pills, desperate and afraid, he quit his job in California and answered an advertisement for a position on the coast of Florida. Even though he had not practiced in Florida for the past ten years, he had kept his medical license in good standing. Despite his troubles in California, he was able to continue working without any questions. He probably thought that perhaps a geographical change would give him the incentive to get clean, but when he arrived he found the problem was even worse.

Within a week of joining the staff at this new hospital, Dr. Thomas was using again. When Ronald arrived for assessment, Dr. Thomas had just taken the last four pills he had. Even though he was feeling high, he knew in the back of his mind that it would only be a matter of hours before the withdrawal began again. After looking over Ronald's chart, he convinced his nurse that Ronald was not having a heart attack but instead needed a prescription for narcotic pain medicine and asked her to bring him the prescription pad for controlled substances. Despite the warning signs that Ronald's condition was not due to a pulled muscle or indigestion, all Dr. Thomas could see was a way to get the pills he needed and wanted. Being high on prescription drugs, he was able to rationalize this behavior and he explained away the concerns that were brought up by the ER nurse. Dr. Thomas wrote a prescription for the narcotics he wanted and, instead of giving it to Ronald, he pocketed the prescription. Then he told the nurse that he had to leave for a few minutes. He knew of a pill mill only a mile or two away that would, for a fee, fill the prescription without any questions asked.

Unfortunately, this scenario is becoming more common. Doctors can do harm with their prescription pads as well as by treating patients while under the influence and Florida is known for its high rate of prescription drug abuse. In 2010, so-called pain clinics in the state were responsible for the distribution of the majority of prescription narcotics in the country, attracting patients (and addicts) from many other states. It's hard to calculate the social costs that result from easy access to these highly addictive medications, but the damage to people and communities is devastating. In Ohio, another state where prescription drug abuse is rampant, overdoses from illicit use of these medications have cost the state an estimated $3.6 billion between 2007 and 2011.[5] People are entering rehabilitation clinics in epidemic numbers, no longer able to afford the prescription medications to which they have become addicted, but these are the lucky ones. Legitimate prescriptions written by physicians for actual patients were responsible for more than fifty overdose-related deaths and one doctor was charged with murder for providing an excessive number of narcotic pain-relieving pills to a patient who died after taking them.

Florida may be the epicenter of the prescription drug addiction epidemic, but its reverberations are felt throughout the United States. According to the 2009 National Survey on Drug Use and Health, almost one third of people who use drugs recreationally for the first time choose to abuse prescription medications.[6] That year, pharmacies dispensed over 257 million prescriptions for opioids, a 47 percent increase from the 174 million prescriptions dispensed just nine years earlier.[7] So prominent has this epidemic become that President Obama called for a response to America's prescription drug abuse crisis. Among the recommendations were a need to increase the education available to both the public and healthcare providers about the dangers of prescription drug abuse, increased utilization of prescription monitoring programs and a legal assault on "pill mills" and "doctor shoppers" who directly contribute to the trafficking of prescription drugs.

Dr. Jeffries, a general practice physician in the Pacific Northwest, wrote over twenty-four different prescriptions for oxycodone and several other highly addictive narcotics over a two-year period for a patient he never actually examined. An investigation by the medical board in the state where he was licensed to practice was sparked when the patient overdosed on the medications he had prescribed for her. The investigation revealed that, despite having written the prescriptions, Dr. Jeffries did not maintain a medical record or list this individual as a patient in his practice. Further investigation revealed that this patient was a prostitute and that the physician had been trading the prescriptions for sex with the woman. The abuse of highly addictive prescription narcotics has reached epidemic proportions in this country and people are willing to do whatever it takes to get their hands on the drugs they need. Physicians are charged with responsibly prescribing potentially dangerous and highly addictive medications and not encouraging their misuse. Behavior such as Dr. Jeffries' only serves to exacerbate the problem.

Another physician, James, himself addicted to prescription narcotics, prescribed medications to his addicted patients in return for sexual favors and with the understanding that they would fill the prescriptions and give him some of the pills. This arrangement was discovered when one of his patients was arrested for a different drug-related offense and "ratted out" the physician in exchange for a lighter sentence.

In another state, Donald, a young pharmacist looking to make a quick buck, was arrested for selling prescription medications out of his car. In the parking lot behind the store where he worked, this recent pharmacy school graduate sold oxycodone, hydrocodone, morphine and other prescription narcotics in wholesale quantities to local dealers for distribution. When the police caught him with a box of controlled drugs in the trunk of his car, he claimed they were for personal use.

Addicted Surgical Technician Exposes Thousands to Virus

Though much less common than the rates seen in anesthesia care providers, anyone with access to drugs used in hospitals has the potential to abuse them. A fair number of surgeons, scrub nurses and surgical technicians, who also work in the same environment, enter treatment for addiction to agents as well. Kristen Parker, a surgical technician, first became addicted to heroin. As a junkie in her home state she shared needles and injection equipment with other addicts and became infected with the hepatitis C virus. Hepatitis C is a nasty virus that slowly destroys the liver. Eventually the infected person will either need a liver transplant or die. Hepatitis C is transmitted through blood and can easily move through populations of drug users if they share injection equipment. Currently, hepatitis C can't be cured; it can be treated, but the success rates are low and the treatment is long and painful. Many patients who start the treatment are unable to complete it because the side effects of the treatment are so debilitating.

Despite her addiction and regular use of heroin, Kristen passed a pre-employment drug screening and obtained a job with access to potent prescription narcotics. As a surgical technician she had access to syringes filled with the much more powerful drug fentanyl. Kristen described how she took these syringes filled with fentanyl and injected herself with the drug before returning the syringes to the operating field, now filled with saline. Still attached were the needles she had used on herself that were contaminated with the hepatitis C virus. Subsequently, these syringes were used on patients receiving surgery, exposing them to the virus. In total, Kristen exposed over six thousand patients to the virus she had and thirty-six patients developed the infection. In February of 2010, Kristen Parker was sentenced to thirty years in prison for this crime, a sentence many have complained is too short given that many of her victims will most likely be dead when she is eventually released.[8]

Stories like those about the addicted physician who traded prescriptions for sex or the pharmacist who ran a drug ring make for sensational newspaper headlines and sound bites for the evening news, but is it possible that these professionals' behavior may be the rule rather than the exception? Is it a real possibility that your health-care provider may also be an addict? Healthcare professionals are just as likely as anyone else to abuse drugs and, as it turns out, more likely to abuse prescription medications. These professionals have ready access to highly addictive controlled medications as well as the intimate knowledge of how these drugs can be safely administered. This combination of access and experience may give some in the medical field the false belief that they can be self-administered with little consequence, but this is not the case and sometimes the results of such behavior can be deadly.

Since the potential for abuse of prescription drugs is so high, how common is drug addiction in this population? Given the rapid decline in addicted healthcare professionals' ability to function, especially when the abused drug is a pharmaceutical with an extremely short half-life such as fentanyl (a narcotic like morphine or heroin, but 100 times more potent), most individuals who are abusing these drugs end up in treatment or dead within a year of having started to use them. If we consider the incidence of admission to a treatment facility as a reflection of the incidence of addiction in a given year, then we can expect that at least 1 to 2 percent of all healthcare professionals will become addicted each year. This data represents only the known cases: cases which come to the attention of the authorities either through the death or respiratory arrest of the individual from overdose, witnessed self-injection or referral to treatment programs. Since not every addicted healthcare professional overdoses, is caught or ends up in a treatment program, the actual number of healthcare professionals diverting medications for personal use is likely much higher. In one recent anonymous survey of healthcare professionals, the numbers were ten times the published results, with as many as 10 to 20 percent of respondents admitting to diverting drugs for personal use.[9] There is a large gap between the reality of the problem and what has been published in the literature.

There is no registry of addicted healthcare professionals to examine and, in the interest of protecting the privacy of addicted individuals, most records of persons who have successfully completed a state-sponsored or private treatment and monitoring program are either sealed or destroyed. Looking closely at state disciplinary actions and mortality statistics can provide further information, but it is hard to put this in context. To use the numbers suggested by these types of reports, one has to assume that all addicted healthcare professionals are reported; this is not the case. Many addicted healthcare professionals do not end up in front of state medical or nursing boards or involved in disciplinary actions. If they do enter treatment, they may do so anonymously and not through a referral from a state agency. As well, since we can't know the total population from which these reported individuals come, we can't generate a percentage, only a raw number. This typically underestimates the scope of the problem.

Because of these issues, the true prevalence of addiction in the population of healthcare professionals remains unknown, though it is reasonable to assume that drug abuse is at least as prevalent in this group of people as it is among the general population. Most studies have found that, at any given moment, 10 to 15 percent of the general population of the United States will meet the criteria for a substance use disorder; that is to say, they will be addicted to some type of drug.[10] Usually this drug is alcohol, but a fair number are also addicted to drugs such as heroin, cocaine, other illicit substances and, more recently, prescription medications. Therefore, since healthcare professionals are at least as likely to become addicted as those in the general population, the prevalence is at least 10 to 15 percent.[11]

Another method for estimating the prevalence of addiction in the population of healthcare workers is through the use of anonymous self-reporting. If we move forward on the assumption that the population of healthcare workers reflects the general population as a whole, it is likely that 10 to 15 percent of all healthcare providers will misuse or abuse drugs or alcohol at some point in their careers. These numbers have been borne out in anonymous surveys which query specific types of healthcare professionals at risk for addiction, such as anesthesia care providers. These surveys ask specific questions about past and present drug use. When currently practicing healthcare professionals answer whether they have ever been addicted to drugs, most who respond report that they are currently in recovery from addiction and that they have been for some time. With striking consistency, most formerly addicted healthcare professionals are open and honest about their histories of addiction. This is probably a reflection of the 12-step philosophy of recovery, which emphasizes honesty and sharing among recovering individuals, to which most recovering healthcare professionals subscribe.

While it may not be surprising that someone who has successfully recovered from addiction is willing to share these details, a much smaller number actually admit to current drug use, either regular casual use or addiction. Since these surveys are aimed at healthcare professionals who are currently in practice, all of the individuals in recovery report being able to return to clinical practice successfully, but disturbingly, the small number who report active use are also in practice. Of the 1 to 2 percent of healthcare workers who become addicted each year, not all of them are able to return to clinical work; in fact, some do not want to. Some choose to practice in nonclinical areas or areas where they are not required to administer controlled substances and some change their professions altogether. A number of physicians and nurses who have been successful in maintaining sobriety through the various recovery programs available to them choose to work in the addiction field, but some give up working in healthcare altogether for fear of relapse.

Another gauge of the prevalence of addiction in this population comes from talking to healthcare professionals who are not addicted or in recovery. If the practice, group or hospital is large enough, it's reasonable to assume that someone is going to take a leave of absence for addiction treatment at some point and it can be very difficult to keep these events confidential. Most healthcare professionals know of one or two people who are in recovery and back at work and a number can tell you stories about people who returned to work only to relapse and lose their licenses. Most of these people are encouraging and supportive about their colleagues' health problems, but not all healthcare workers feel positive about the prospect for treatment when it comes to issues related to addiction.

David, a nurse who works in the intensive care unit at a hospital in California, states, "When people go away for a while and then when they come back they can't handle the narcotics, it's pretty clear what's going on. By the end of their first shifts back everyone who is there knows what's going on and by the next day the whole unit knows. I know we're supposed to respect these people's confidentiality, but that's just the way it is. If a nurse didn't want to be talked about, she shouldn't have started using drugs in the first place."

David's resentment toward his colleagues in recovery is clear. "The reality is that I have enough work to do myself without having to do their work too. If they can't pull their own weight, they shouldn't be here." It is precisely because of this attitude or the fear that they may be met with resistance or resentment that many healthcare professionals in recovery, who wish to return to work after treatment, are tempted to try to keep their recoveries to themselves. However, as we will see, the basis for successful recovery depends upon open and honest accountability. Not allowing affected individuals the opportunity to take responsibility for their actions within a climate of care and concern can have disastrous consequences.

CHAPTER 3

How Could This Affect Me?

T he disease of addiction is so powerful that otherwise reasonable and intelligent people often resort to unscrupulous behavior in order to obtain their drugs of choice. The need for
drugs is so strong that addicted healthcare professionals no longer
place the needs of their patients before their own. Addicted physicians and nurses who are more concerned with how they are going
to get their next fixes cannot provide adequate healthcare, which is
exactly why you should worry about how an addicted healthcare
professional could personally affect your health and well-being.

Mountain Climber, Adrenaline Junkie and Dope Fiend

Doug was formally trained as an emergency medicine physician and
worked for several years in a busy emergency department in a hospital located in the Northeast before he developed an addiction to
prescription narcotics. When I met him he was a patient at a facility
that specializes in the treatment of addicted healthcare professionals.
Doug's story is typical of the emergency medicine physicians who
become addicted to prescription medications. "I've always been an
adrenaline junkie, skydiving, mountain climbing, ironman competi-
tions, you name it. For me it wasn't the need to get high as much as
the need to slow down. I had so much internal energy it was hard
to turn it off, to be able to decompress." Doug had access to a wide
range of prescription medications, but taking them from hospital

supplies in the quantities he needed would arouse suspicion, so he came up with another way to obtain the drugs he wanted.

"We all had access to each other's prescription pads," he explained. "They were locked up, but if a nurse needed to write a script for a patient she could take one and then the doc would just sign it. I didn't want anyone to be able to trace these scripts back to me, so I took scripts from the other docs and forged their signatures. Then I wrote the script out for thirty oxycodone tablets or whatever I needed with no refills (so as not to arouse suspicion) and used the name of a patient who came into the ER that day. The names were real, so if anyone did crosscheck, I figured it would check out. I mean, these were real people who actually were patients at my hospital and the scripts were from ER docs who worked at the hospital, so how could I get caught?" As Doug explained this to me there was no hint that he fully comprehended how his actions could have possibly harmed anyone but himself. Practicing emergency medicine while under the influence of prescription narcotics increased the risk that he might miss an important diagnosis or make an error on a procedure. It put every one of his patients at risk for serious harm. Using the names of his patients to obtain prescriptions illegally for his own personal use could have also impacted these people. Forging his colleagues' names on their prescription pads could have destroyed others' careers as well as his own. "Just to be sure I wasn't recognized," he revealed, "I always wore dark glasses and a hat when I presented the scripts to the pharmacy, I used the drive-through windows at drugstores whenever possible and I never went to the same place twice."

Despite his well-thought-out plans, Doug was eventually caught. "By the time I realized I had become addicted I couldn't stop. I needed so many pills just to prevent the withdrawal symptoms, just to feel normal, that I got sloppy." Apparently a suspicious pharmacist called the Drug Enforcement Agency (DEA) and they conducted an investigation. "An agent showed up at work one day with a photo of me, apparently taken by a security camera at one of the drive-through pharmacies, asking if anyone knew who I was. They had apparently traced the scripts back to my ER, but they assumed I was a patient, not an ER doc. I was arrested at gunpoint in the parking lot of the hospital and taken to jail. They found so many pills in my locker at work that they charged me with distribution. They said there was no way that anyone would need that many pills for personal use. They charged me with a felony. The only reason I'm in treatment and not in jail is because of my lawyer, but he says there's a good chance I'll lose my license anyway. I may never be able to practice medicine again."

Anesthesiologist Kept Drugs for Himself

Can you imagine waking up from surgery having received little or no pain medications? Sometimes, instead of stealing medications using a patient's name, addicted healthcare professionals will steal the medications directly from the patients. An anesthesia care provider who is addicted may indicate in the medical record that a narcotic was given to a patient during surgery when in fact the provider kept the narcotic for himself and administered either an alternate agent or none at all. Todd, an anesthesiologist, was admitted to the same facility as Doug after he injected himself with what he though was fentanyl but turned out to be a paralytic agent, then collapsed during surgery and had to be resuscitated by the operating room staff. Todd openly described his behavior, which resulted in patient harm. "I had placed an intravenous (IV) line in a vein in my leg and taped the catheter so the injection port rested just below the top of the boots I wore while at work," Todd revealed. "All I had to do was reach down like I was pulling up my socks or something and inject a little fentanyl and I was good to go. Every time I gave some to a patient I split the dose so we each got some, but of course I charted all of the fentanyl as given to the patient. That's how it started out, but it wasn't long, maybe a couple weeks, maybe a month, before I was using so much that I needed to keep all the fentanyl for myself."

Fentanyl has a relatively short half-life and tolerance can develop rapidly. It is not uncommon for an addict in recovery to report self-administration of 1,000 micrograms of fentanyl in a single injection, often simply to relieve the symptoms of withdrawal. For comparison, a typical medical case involving general anesthesia may involve only 250 micrograms of fentanyl, an amount which will stop most people from breathing. To obtain this quantity of fentanyl to meet the body's increasing needs, an addicted healthcare professional must steal more and more of the drug. The records of addicted anesthesiologists will likely show an increased quantity of narcotics used, particularly on Fridays, when they have to prepare for a weekend away from their sources. Todd went on to state: "I did entire cases without giving the patient any pain medicine. I used other drugs to keep patients' heart rates and blood pressures down so they wouldn't look like they needed any pain medication, but I wrote in the charts that I had administered the narcotics so I could keep them for myself. I can't believe I actually did these things, but I wasn't thinking about the patient on the table or about losing my job or even about what might happen to me if anyone ever found out. All I cared about was getting enough fentanyl for my next fix."

But it wasn't just the patients he was taking care of that Todd put at risk. "Whenever I was assigned to give coffee breaks to my colleagues I took the fentanyl they had already drawn up for the cases they were doing and substituted syringes with some other drug. It's all clear liquid anyway, so there's no way to tell what's really in the syringe. You have to go by what's on the label." With this deception, for example, when an anesthesiologist whom Todd had relieved returned from his break, there would be no way for him to know that the clear liquid in the syringe labeled "fentanyl" was not actually a narcotic. Later, when the heart rate of the patient under anesthesia began to increase, suggesting the fentanyl was wearing off, the anesthesiologist would administer what was in the syringe, thinking that he was treating the patient's pain appropriately. If Todd had substituted a drug which would slow the patient's heart rate for the fentanyl he had taken for himself, then the decrease in the patient's heart rate might even be as expected if a narcotic was administered. But later, at the end of the surgery, this patient would likely wake up in pain well out of proportion to the amount of narcotics he or she had supposedly been given.

Because addicted health professionals can't always depend on patient cases having the drugs they need, they quickly become proficient at removing controlled substances from secure places. The security features of automated dispensing machines are easily defeated and dispensing records are rarely crosschecked with patient records on a regular basis. Despite the increased security touted by the manufacturers of the automated devices that dispense controlled substances throughout hospitals, formerly addicted healthcare professionals consistently report being able to obtain their drugs of choice easily from these machines without getting caught. One particularly cocky individual used to refer to the device where he used to work as the "vending machine."

Not all addicts have their own personal narcotic vending machines, however, and some must resort to other means of obtaining their drugs. "Sometimes if we don't have the right label for a particular drug, we substitute a different label," Todd explained. "Or sometimes we may reuse a syringe with a narcotic label to draw up another drug so there's no guarantee that the syringe you're taking actually has fentanyl in it and that's so dangerous, but you wouldn't believe the things addicts have to do just to avoid withdrawal." This is how Todd was discovered. During a relief break he rummaged through the sharps waste containers in the operating rooms, looking for residual drugs in discarded syringes. He found a syringe labeled "fentanyl" and took it back to his operating room. Once the anesthesiologist who had given him the break was gone, Todd injected the liquid into his leg. "I immediately knew something was wrong. I didn't feel the rush that I always felt when I injected fentanyl. I figured it was just a flush (a volume of inert liquid, usually saline, used to push other drugs through the intravenous line and into the patient) that someone had discarded, but then I started to get weak."

Todd realized that he had given himself an injection of a paralytic agent, but there was nothing he could do. "Within seconds I slid out of the chair I was sitting in and fell flat on my face. I was totally awake and aware of what was going on. For what seemed like an eternity, I thought that nobody would notice and I would suffocate there on the floor, unable to breathe, while the surgery continued." Luckily for Todd, the circulating nurse did notice that he was no longer in his position at the head of the bed. She and an attendant walked over to investigate.

"They rolled me over and checked for a pulse," Todd described. "I could hear them talking, but I couldn't tell them what was happening. They called for help and an anesthesiologist from another room came in and placed a breathing tube in my trachea. I was placed on a ventilator, since I was paralyzed and couldn't breathe on my own, and transferred to the intensive care unit for observation. It was only a short while before they found the intravenous in my leg and figured out what had happened, but they thought I had overdosed on narcotics. When the paralytic wore off, they removed the breathing tube and I was able to explain what happened. That afternoon they transferred me to a treatment center."

If Todd had not been discovered facedown at the head of the bed, he may not have been the only person to die that day. As an anesthesiologist, Todd's primary function is keeping the patient alive, asleep and pain-free during the surgery. There's no telling what might have happened if nobody had noticed he was missing from his post.

Jaded, Faded Junkie Nurse

It is not only physicians who are involved with the diversion of controlled substances for personal use. Kristen, a registered nurse who used to work in a pediatric intensive care unit, described how she took morphine or hydromorphone intended for her patients and used it herself. "These babies were all so tiny; the amount of each drug they got was just a small part of what the syringes held. We got the drugs in standard concentrations and then had to dilute them down to be able to give appropriate doses to the patients. It seemed such a shame to waste what was left over." Kristen started keeping the leftovers for herself. Nurses are supposed to witness colleagues' disposing controlled substances, but as Kristen pointed out, "They never knew that I had removed the morphine and replaced it with saline." Since they weren't required to return the leftover narcotics to the pharmacy for testing, she wasn't caught until a suspicious colleague reported her behavior as suspect.

To behave in a way that goes directly against the moral compass of most healthcare professionals requires performing these acts in secret. While this behavior may seem unimaginable to some, the drive to obtain the drug of choice is so strong that addicts must suspend their sense of right and wrong. As incredible as it may seem, it is likely that stories such as Kristen's represent only the tip of the iceberg, so to speak, and more disturbing behavior is revealed only during therapy sessions or private conversations in closed-door meetings with other addicted healthcare professionals.

Collateral Damage

When a healthcare professional becomes addicted to alcohol or drugs, it is not just his or her patients who have the potential to be harmed. Often, these people are the primary providers of their households' incomes. The loss of these resources for extended periods of time coupled with the high costs of treatment can devastate families financially. The other spouse may have to return to work or work a second job; children may have to leave private schools or forgo extracurricular activities, possibly even quitting afterschool activities to take on jobs to help support the family.

For physicians or advanced practice nurses with higher salaries, vacations, new cars, clothes and all of the trappings of upper-middle class life quickly fade into the past as resources are funneled toward treatment, monitoring and legal defense. Relations with colleagues or other peers in the community may become strained as the retreat from social or public life becomes apparent. Financial stress on top of what is almost always an emotionally stressful time in the months or years leading up to and during treatment can cause separation or divorce for some couples.

To survive both addiction and recovery requires a strong partner, someone willing to forgive past behaviors, accept responsibility for any enabling or codependent behavior and accept the dramatic changes that come with recovery. Many relationships are not this strong and many couples don't make it through the first year. Those that do will likely find that the relationship dynamic has been forever altered by the experience, hopefully for the better.

Brian and Emily are one couple who were able to survive Brian's addiction to fentanyl and subsequent treatment, but it was not an easy road to recovery. "I began using fentanyl as an anesthesia resident," Brian explained, "mostly to manage my mood during the long and sometimes stressful days. When I was using, I felt like I had so much energy and nothing seemed to bother me. Our residency program is so malignant and it was the only way I could deal with the constant berating from my attending physicians. It seemed like I could do nothing the right way, but when I was using then the verbal abuse was easier to take."

But it wasn't just stress on the job that led to Brian's fentanyl use; things at home had also become difficult. "Emily got very sick during the first year of my training and she couldn't work anymore, so we were entirely dependent on my salary. Residents aren't paid a whole lot of money and I had to support my wife and our young son and cover the mortgage on the new house we had just bought. This was a lot of financial pressure." It seems the pressure both at work and at home was too much for Brian and he chose to abuse fentanyl to deal with it. "I was hooked within a week and three months later I was a complete and total wreck."

Emily could tell that something terribly wrong was happening to Brian, but she had no clue what was going on. "He often came home late; he was always in a bear of a mood. He became so short-tempered and nasty that I used to cringe when I heard him come through the front door. Eventually I began to hope he would never come home at all." It was only a matter of time before Brian's fentanyl diversion was discovered and Emily finally got her wish one late winter afternoon. "I got a call from Brian's program director, a man I knew by name but had never met. He told me what Brian had been doing and said that Brian would be going away for a while. I immediately exhaled a sigh of relief."

Brian described their continued financial troubles: "When I was caught, they sent me to an inpatient rehab program for twelve weeks. My insurance covered the first ten days, then I had to make up the difference. The place they sent me charged $4,000 a week. The only way we could pay for this was to charge the bill on our credit cards. When I completed the program I found out that I had been dismissed from my residency program. So there I was, with no job, no health insurance, a $40,000 credit card bill for treatment, a mortgage payment and a family to support. On top of that, the hospital that I had worked for had reported my case to the medical board, so there was an investigation and I had to hire a lawyer, which cost me another $10,000 up front and the physician health program I had signed a contract with mandated that I see a psychiatrist twice a week."

Soon the hard economic reality of their situation began to dawn on Emily. "I had no idea that this would completely devastate us financially. Three weeks into Brian's treatment I was just getting over being mad as hell that he had left me to take care of our son and run the house all alone when he told me about the insurance coverage issue." Emily and Brian had no savings to fall back on. "We had taken a cash advance on one of our credit cards to make up the difference between what we had and what we needed for the down payment on the new house, so all of our money was tied up in there. We had only been in the house for nine months when Brian left for treatment, so all I could do was triage the bills and pay the most essential ones. At one point I was using cash advance checks from one credit card to pay the minimum payment on a card from a different company."

The irony that Brian's choice of using fentanyl to deal with the financial pressure he was feeling exponentially increased this financial pressure was not lost on Emily. "Brian took a bad situation and made it worse, so much worse," she reflected.

Brian and Emily were able to float for a while using the credit they had established over the years. "This was before the recession, back when credit was much more available. I remember one night Brian and I sat on the bed and took out all our cards and figured out we had something like $300,000 in available credit and offers kept coming in the mail. I don't know what we would do in these times; as it is, we can barely make the monthly bills."

Once Brian was discharged and returned home, things got worse. "It seemed like our debt just continued to snowball. Not only did I no longer have a job but also I had to attend meetings every day and individual or group therapy twice a week, so it was hard to find a new job. I couldn't work in anything related to healthcare as mandated by my monitoring contract and I kept thinking it would only be a few short months before I could resume my training."

The psychiatrist to whom Brian was referred apparently had been left with unpaid bills by some physician patients before. "He had a credit card machine in his office and before each session he swiped my card to get payment. For the group sessions he swiped everyone's card before starting the session. It was like this bizarre ritual, which would have been amusing if I had any idea how I was going to be able to pay for it."

Emily had her own problems to deal with as well. "I started noticing that my 'friends' weren't coming around much anymore. At first they asked why I wasn't at a particular event or why Brian and I hadn't attended the gala for such-and-such a charity, but then they started to gossip and I discovered most of those people really weren't my friends. I told myself that I was more upset for our son, who didn't get to see his friends when their mommies didn't bring them around, but he was young at the time and it was more about how hurt I was."

The treatment and monitoring process for a physician can involve a long time away from work and, with limited financial resources, it can be extremely difficult to keep up the façade that everything is alright. "Brian and I worked so hard for that house; it was all we had in this world. I'd be damned if I was going to let it go without a fight."

With more free time than Brian knew what to do with and a need to come up with enough cash to pay the mortgage and essential monthly bills until he could find another job, Brian set out to try to bring in some income. "I had some experience selling things online in the past, so I figured it might be a good way to make some quick cash." Brian started with the things they already had. "I went into the garage, the basement, the attic, anywhere we might have things we weren't using. I figured if we hadn't used it since I went away for treatment then we could do just fine without it. I couldn't believe how much stuff we had managed to accumulate in such a short period of time." Brian spent hours every day photographing and then writing detailed listings for everything he found. "If you take a nice photo and write a catchy description, people will pay for almost anything. I even sold a lot of used (but washed) baby socks and I got five dollars for them!" Brian says that at one point he had over 150 seven-day auctions running. "I didn't care if it was a ninety-nine-cent item or a ninety-nine-dollar one. Every little bit I could bring in was needed." When the storage spaces were empty he took all the things that didn't sell online and had a garage sale. "I was surprised what people were willing to pay for what I considered at this point to be mostly junk. I didn't make a lot of cash at that garage sale, but it got me thinking." That evening Brian and Emily took a drive around their neighborhood. "It was early in the summer and our neighbors were also having garage sales. That night, after it got dark, we drove through the streets looking for discarded items that hadn't sold at the day's sales. We picked through the 'trash' at our neighbors' curbs and took anything I thought that I might be able to clean up and then sell." For the rest of the summer, sifting through their neighbors' discarded items became ritual for the couple. "You know, what they say is actually true: one man's trash really is another man's treasure."

Despite the abundance of discarded items to pick up and sell, Brian was unable to make enough to cover the monthly bills without also selling some higher end items. "It was hard when I had to start selling Emily's jewelry, but we both knew we had to sell everything we owned or lose the house." Shoes, clothes and designer pocketbooks followed until there was very little left. "In some ways it was very liberating," Emily revealed. "It was as if we were a team again, working as hard as we could to keep our heads above water. But then I would think about the necklace that Brian had bought for me that was now hanging around some stranger's neck and I would start to get mad again." Emily also lost a friend who discovered a gift she had given Emily was up for auction. "I couldn't tell my friend the situation we were in. I was so ashamed and she just stopped talking to me after that. It was mortifying."

Things are different now for Brian and Emily. It has been nine years since Brian entered treatment and he is now working as an attending anesthesiologist. "Eventually I was allowed to return to finish my training and I graduated from residency five years ago." Despite a full-time job with an impressive salary in the mid six figures, the financial fallout from the eighteen months Brian was out of work is still with them. "We are still paying off the credit card bills we ran up and we still have my student loans and our mortgage." After taxes, Brian now brings home enough to cover the minimum payments on their almost $275,000 credit card debt and $175,000 medical school loans as well as the mortgage on their house, the home they wanted so desperately to keep. Even though things are still tight, there is an end they both can foresee. "I figure we'll be done with the credit cards in about ten more years and then things will start to get easier. At least we didn't have to file bankruptcy. That was important to both of us."

Emily has also learned to live with the changes. "I care much less now about superficial things. I still really appreciate fine jewelry, couture clothes and designer shoes, but I'm (usually) able to keep things in perspective. I have a small group of really good friends who know what we've been through and understand. I don't think I would have found such good people if I hadn't gone through this with Brian. Not only is our relationship that much stronger, but also so are the relationships I have with my 'real' friends and the family members who stood by us when it looked like we might lose everything."

A life crisis of this magnitude can shift the very foundations of a relationship. If we recognize the need to make changes in the way we deal with those around us and work hard, we can use this crisis as an opportunity and come through not only having survived, but also having changed for the better. Brian and Emily were able to survive Brian's addiction to fentanyl and subsequent treatment, because they were both committed to each other and not to the material things they had accumulated or to the status they had achieved. By being able to let go of material and somewhat unimportant things and focus on the common goal of keeping their family together, they were able to succeed.

Realizing Codependency

Not every couple, however, is either as motivated or as capable of such effort as Brian and Emily demonstrated. For some, one spouse's descent into addiction is just another item in a long list of problems the couple has encountered and it becomes an excuse to part ways. For others, it is the recovery itself that presents the problem. No longer in the dependent role, the recovering partner may find that his spouse is no longer comfortable with him or with their relationship. The codependent spouse, realizing that the relationship dynamic has now changed considerably, may become angry with the partner who is in recovery. At that point, either partner may decide to end the relationship or, worse, fall back into the old comfortable roles of addict and enabler.

Mike and Lisa had only been married for a year before Lisa entered treatment for addiction to prescription painkillers. "I had been working as an advanced practice nurse in a rural area in Iowa as part of my payback to the National Health Service for covering my student loans. I was so far out in the middle of nowhere that I basically ran the practice myself. The family physician who supervised the practice came by once a week and to see any follow-up patients with particularly complicated issues, but I took care of all of the bread and butter stuff myself." Lisa was not originally from the Midwest and the lifestyle was not what she was used to. "I moved here from a city on the East Coast. There's a lot to do in a city that size; here, not so much."

Lisa worked five days a week and then returned to the East Coast to be with her husband on the weekends. "It was rough, but it was only going to be for two years and we both decided that it would be better than having to pay the loans off ourselves." For the first year the arrangement seemed to work, but the distance was far and while Mike had his friends and family with him at their home, Lisa was all alone. "I started taking the oxycodone or whatever we had in the practice just to keep up the energy, to keep going during the day and to drive off the boredom after work. I had no idea I was becoming addicted."

Weekly trips home became more expensive and after a while Lisa returned only once or twice a month. "My schedule became unpredictable and one Friday I showed up at home late in the evening to find Mike in bed with one of our friends. In retrospect it was obvious that something like that was going to happen—you can't spend that much time apart in a marriage and expect to stay together—but I really didn't expect him to cheat on me with another man."

Lisa says that walking in on her husband and another man having sex was the jolt she needed to make some major changes in her life. Ironically, though, it wasn't Lisa who asked Mike for a divorce. "After our 'friend' left, we spent the weekend talking about our relationship. When I told him what I had been doing and that I was addicted to prescription medications, he said that was too much for him and he wanted to get divorced. To this day, I don't believe he's gay and if I hadn't walked in on them I bet we would still be together."

Lisa left her position at the family practice clinic in Iowa and entered treatment for her addiction. "We got a quick divorce. It was finalized after I was discharged from treatment, but Mike was gone by then."

Even though Mike did not want to talk with Lisa, he agreed to talk with me about his decision to leave their marriage. "I was still mad at her for leaving me and going to Iowa," he explained. "This was *her* decision, something *she* wanted to do. She made it seem like this was something we both wanted to do, spend the first years of our marriage apart, but that's how Lisa is." Two years after the separation, Mike still sounds resentful. "I had already checked out. Her addiction was just an excuse to leave."

Sometimes, however, the spouses of addicted healthcare professionals don't have the luxury of considering whether or not to keep the family together. Sometimes the decision is made for them in the moments after a fatal overdose claims the lives of their loved ones. Despite the impressive success rates boasted by today's addiction treatment programs aimed at rehabilitating addicted healthcare professionals, some never make it into treatment to begin with. The prescription medications available today are so powerful that a minor miscalculation in dose can mean the difference between life and death.

A number of physicians, nurses and other healthcare professionals with access to prescription medications overdose on them and die each year. These people are not included in the statistics that claim a successful treatment rate better than twice that of what the civilian programs claim to offer; their numbers can be found in the mortality statistics, often by sifting through autopsy records of patients with noncommittal "cardiovascular disease" listed as the cause of death. Was the physician found alone with evidence suggesting self-administration of a controlled substance? Was there a syringe containing traces of a drug at his side? Did the blood from his veins test positive for that same drug? Many of these deaths are never properly classified as the result of addiction to prescription medications, but when a young person dies and the cause of death is conspicuously absent from the obituary, I can't help but wonder.

Addicted healthcare professionals are unable to provide the high quality care that we desire, need and expect, despite their best intentions or their beliefs that somehow being high doesn't interfere with their ability to practice medicine. As we have seen, this can negatively impact you, the healthcare consumer, in many different ways, some of which are more subtle than others. An intoxicated physician who is performing a procedure or monitoring your vital signs while under anesthesia presents a clear and present danger, but what about the distracted healthcare professional who is more concerned with where he will get his next fix? In the hectic pace of today's healthcare environment, even the smallest mistake or oversight has the potential for dire consequences.

The disease of addiction not only affects the careers of highly educated professionals with considerable promise and puts their patients at profound risk, but also can destroy the families of these professionals. The people who depend on these addicted healthcare professionals for support, financial and otherwise, may find themselves having to support the former breadwinner and many marriages have not survived this significant stress.

What about an addicted healthcare professional who is able to enter treatment? Even those who successfully enter the specialized treatment programs that are available for addicted healthcare professionals are not guaranteed success. Some addicts simply cannot stay clean, no matter what treatment they receive. Others may think they can take "just one more shot" and end up self-administering a dose of the drug far in excess of what would kill someone with no tolerance. It is not known how many of these so-called "hot shots" are responsible for the deaths of addicted healthcare professionals in recovery each year, but talking to the surviving family members does shed some light on the struggles that the addicted professionals go through.

PART II

HOW HEALTHCARE PROFESSIONALS BECOME ADDICTED

CHAPTER 4

The Origins of Addiction

H ealthcare professionals are members of the general population long before they become members of the subpopulation of healthcare workers. Some may have developed addictions to drugs before or during the course of their professional educations and may begin their medical careers either actively addicted or in recovery. For those who become addicted to drugs after beginning work in the healthcare field, it is likely that the same predispositions to the development of addiction found in the general population play a role and, in some cases, may actually influence career choice.

Sex, Drugs and Nursing

Michelle, a nurse in recovery from addiction to prescription medications, revealed that both her addiction and her recovery predated her medical training. "I actually started using long before I was a nurse." Attractive, socially competent and a good student, Michelle seemed like she had it all, but under the thin veneer she presented to the world lay a very different person. "I was always angry and easily annoyed, but I kept all of this to myself."

Unlike most teenagers who act out a lot, Michelle felt unable to express outwardly her disgust for the people around her. "I did a lot of things just to buck authority; things that I knew would annoy my family and sometimes my friends. If there was a rule then I broke it, just because it was there, and I felt most rules were stupid anyway." The idea that society's rules apply to others and not the individual is not a new concept. Most teenagers have felt this way at one time or another and many have acted upon their feelings, but this persistent belief that Michelle had that she was somehow different from everybody else allowed her to engage in behaviors that grew increasingly dangerous.

Introduced to alcohol by a friend at a party, Michelle's early experience is typical of many addicts who begin to drink before they are twenty-one. "I first started drinking alcohol when I was thirteen years old. The first time I drank I had a total blackout. I was always uncomfortable in my own skin and I loved the way liquor made me feel." Alcohol is the most common drug abused by members of our society, regardless of age or profession. Many healthcare professionals in recovery from addiction to prescription medications report starting with alcohol long before gaining access to the medications that eventually put them in treatment.

Despite laws which currently make it illegal for persons in the United States under the age of twenty-one to purchase beverages containing alcohol, restricted access remains an easily overcome formality. "When I was in high school," Michelle related, "there was a liquor store not far from my house. They sold to anyone with cash." Easy access to alcohol is a contributing factor to underage use, but even if the majority of teenagers will try alcohol at some point in their development, most of these young people will not become alcoholics. While most people report some experience with alcohol before turning twenty-one, the majority of these people do not regularly drink to blackout. However, drinking to excess in order to escape feelings of inadequacy or anxiety is a common theme reported by alcoholics and addicts with a history of alcohol abuse.

"The summer that I turned thirteen was not only my first experience with alcohol, but it was also the year I started having sex," Michelle divulged. Even if 50 percent of girls in the mid-1990s reported having sexual intercourse by the time they turned eighteen years old, only 8 percent reported doing so before age fourteen.[1] Michelle may have started having sex much earlier than other teenagers in her peer group due to her alcohol use. "We partied with the junior and senior kids and there was always an older boy who was happy to have a wasted freshman girl at the party. I got drunk and let them do whatever they wanted. I did it because I knew enough to know better. I knew that good kids weren't supposed to behave like this and since it was 'against the rules' to have sex, that's what I did."

Michelle regularly drove a car while under the influence, ignored speed restrictions and basic traffic laws, continued to have unprotected sex and drank heavily throughout high school. The fact that she never got caught or had to pay any consequences for her behavior reinforced her perception of herself as somehow different and more privileged than anyone else. "I began to think of myself as a cat, you know, with nine lives. I tried to push the envelope as far as I could just to see if I could rip it open. I took any drug that was available: marijuana, cocaine, methamphetamines, ecstasy. If I could smoke it, snort it or swallow it to get high, I did. I went to school with a tab of acid under my tongue and spent the day tripping. I brought in a bottle of vodka and mixed it in a cup with orange juice and drank it right in front of my teachers. There are so many times I should have crashed my car, gotten pregnant, contracted a sexually transmitted disease or choked to death on my own vomit in my friend's backyard because I'd had too much to drink, but none of that ever happened."

Individuals who are at greater risk for developing the disease of addiction typically exhibit traits such as "novelty seeking," "sensation seeking" and "antisocial behavior" before they become addicts. Many have been diagnosed with oppositional defiant disorder or exhibit behaviors such as a disregard for authority or anger and frustration with those around them. These people may seek new and different experiences, be more willing to try something new or think outside the box. Rarely, these people are involved with criminal behaviors unrelated to drug use, such as robbery and other violent crimes. Individuals with these traits may choose fields which provide the stimulation that they seek or may choose to abuse drugs when these sensations are lacking from their daily lives. There appears to be a genetic basis for both the development of these traits and the susceptibility to dependence on drugs. Often, more than one person in a particular family has these issues.

By the time Michelle was in college, she had found substances she liked even better than alcohol or street drugs. "The first time I diverted medications was during nursing school when I was working at a pharmacy. I took whatever I could get my hands on, but ultimately I fell in love with narcotic pain relievers and the combination of acetaminophen, butalbital and caffeine, which is supposed to be for headaches. Since I had worked in the pharmacy for so long, I was already educated regarding what *should* be controlled but was not." Michelle discovered that drugs with profound effects on mood like butalbital, nalbuphine and butorphanol were not controlled substances.

"When I started working in the hospital and reading the package inserts, I recall thinking, 'This stuff should be locked up because people like me will take it!' I knew what these drugs could do, so I took them." Although Michelle feels she would have become addicted to just about anything, free access to these mood-altering drugs played a role in her choice of prescription medications as the drugs she abused. "In the pharmacy we used to throw away broken pills! I knew I could skim off the top and nobody would know."

Even though becoming a nurse requires a significant amount of education, very little of it is focused on addiction, just as in medical school, and none on the problem of addiction in healthcare providers. "We had one lecture on street drugs that your patients might have taken and of course we learned the signs and symptoms of withdrawal and what to do about it, but nobody ever said anything about nurses who use these drugs on themselves. I thought that was odd, because my first thought was about how I could get these good drugs for myself, but I was glad that nobody else knew what signs and symptoms to look for." Michelle figured that if her colleagues weren't being trained on what to look for in nurses who were abusing, then she had a better chance of not being caught.

With a significant history of drug abuse and personality characteristics suggestive of oppositional defiant disorder, Michelle began her career as a nurse. Working in a busy acute care unit, she took care of mostly elderly patients with multiple medical problems. "The patients I cared for were really sick and sometimes they had me cover three or four patients at a time, because we were so understaffed. I didn't mind, because it just gave me more opportunities to divert the drugs I needed." In the course of a twelve-hour shift, Michelle was charged with administering medications to each of her patients on a regular schedule. "Most of them were on some sort of narcotic and, even if they only had an as-needed order, I could still sign the pills out under their names." If there was any question about what she was doing or if a patient's family was there, substituting an uncontrolled drug like acetaminophen or ibuprofen for the narcotics she wanted gave the appearance that she was actually giving the medicine to her patients. In fact, Michelle was diverting the narcotics for her own personal use. "I was constantly high. I took most of the pills as soon as I got them, because it was safer than having them on me. But I had to make sure there were enough to make it through the evenings and the days when I wasn't at work."

There is no question that her behavior put her patients at significant risk and may have resulted in harm. "As a nurse, I am supposed to be the one watching the patients for signs of trouble. In addition to taking care of their daily needs like food and medications, I need to be able to identify trends in vital signs or levels of consciousness and intervene before it's too late. It's impossible to maintain that level of vigilance when you're high on pills."

Michelle was able to rationalize her behavior, because she really believed that she was somehow different from everyone else who had ever taken drugs. "At first I was convinced that I could take these pills and nothing bad would ever happen, to me or anyone else. I was a superwoman. Other people got addicted to drugs; I was above that. I believed I worked better when I was high and I felt more alert and less edgy, so I told myself that my patients were getting the best 'Nurse Michelle' they could when I had taken their medication myself. By the time it was obvious to me that I was completely and totally addicted to this stuff, I told myself that because I was different, because I was special, it didn't matter. I needed drugs to feel normal and when I was normal I could be a good nurse." When she was high Michelle felt better but she didn't perform better and people started to notice.

Other nurses and the doctors on the unit began to wonder why Michelle's patients seemed to require so much more pain medication, yet always complained of being in pain. Instead of focusing on completing the demanding workload before the end of the shift, Michelle focused on how she was going to get enough drugs to make it through the off hours when she was away from the hospital. Her colleagues began to resent having to pick up her patients at the end of her shift because she always left so much undone.

Eventually someone said something, but not directly to her. Michelle says that the intervention did not go well at all. "My intervention sucked; it was botched. I was confronted with plenty of evidence, which of course I denied. I was so deathly afraid of losing my supply; I didn't give a crap about anything else. I was so addicted and so sick." The people who confronted Michelle offered her help if she would only admit that she had a problem. "Of course I continued to deny it. I was so scared." With that, her supervisor slid a pen and a piece of paper across the table and asked her to write her letter of resignation.

"They let me drive home. I was high as a kite. I was also suicidal. Thank goodness I didn't have the guts to do it. I didn't know who would take care of my pets and that stopped me from doing anything stupid." The fact that an overdose or other drug-related incident would have the same result of orphaning her dogs seemed lost on her at that time. "I did not want to live. I knew the drugs were killing me, but I could not imagine my life without them. I should never have been left alone."

Shortly after her intervention, detectives started calling her house. Faced with the knowledge that she would likely have to face criminal charges and not wanting to go through withdrawal in jail, Michelle chose to try to get off narcotics at home.

Eight hours after her last pill, Michelle began to feel restless. She began to sweat, her eyes began to tear and her nose began to run. "At first it was like a really bad cold." But within hours the cold had turned into a flu-like syndrome and she was balled up on her couch shaking under several layers of blankets. "The heat was on eighty degrees and I was fully clothed under a thick pile of blankets and I could not get warm. It was horribly unpleasant. It sucked. I couldn't sleep, everything ached and I was miserable. All I wanted was more drugs." In an attempt to mitigate the effects of withdrawal, Michelle drank alcohol and smoked marijuana. "It was all I had and it didn't work well at all."

Michelle spent the following week alone in her apartment, suffering through the acute withdrawal phase of her recovery. "By the time I was done I would have been happy to die." Though rarely fatal, withdrawal can be subjectively very distressing and avoidance of these symptoms may be the primary reason addicts continue to use, despite receiving no other benefit from opioid use and in the face of significant negative consequences. "Even though you know trying to get just one more fix may get you caught or thrown in jail, when you're going through this all you can think is 'I know how to make it stop' and most people can't do it on their own."

The Junkie Who Treats Junkies

Kramer never seemed satisfied with his life; nothing was ever good enough. "I was always an anxious person. I felt like nothing I ever did was as good as it could be and I blamed most of my problems on other people." He chose to become a radiologist not because he wanted to, but because it seemed like a low-stress alternative to the other medical specialties. But even healthcare professions you might not consider stressful by nature can be, given the right combination of personality and job dissatisfaction. Unfortunately, his combination of undiagnosed mental illness and easy access to highly addictive prescription medications eventually caused Kramer's world to come crashing down around him like some self-fulfilling prophecy.

Growing up the eldest son of two professional parents who were rarely home, Kramer had much of the responsibility for caring for his two younger siblings. "From a very early age I was in charge. I made sure my brother and sister got off to school in the morning. I made us breakfast and packed our lunches. After school I made sure we all got our homework done before watching television." By the time he was in fifth grade Kramer knew he wanted to join the military. "I loved the idea of having to make your bed so perfect, with the sheets and blanket tucked in so tight you could bounce a quarter off it. I guess the combination of high expectations and rigorous routine appealed to me. I needed to know what was expected of me." Despite eventually pursuing a career in medicine, his dream of going to boot camp never died and Kramer joined the Navy after graduating from medical school.

Kramer recalled, "I first noticed that prescription medications could alleviate my stress and help me cope with my feelings during the first year of my residency, but it didn't really escalate until two years later. I have always been anxious and somewhat depressed, but I never bothered to see a psychiatrist or even talk to another doctor about what to do. I am prone to getting migraine headaches and when I took butalbital I always felt better." Addiction rarely develops in a vacuum. Often there is coexisting mental illness, typically in the form of depression, anxiety or personality disorders, which exist prior to the development of drug dependence. Healthcare professionals develop the same range of emotional and psychiatric problems as the general population, with the exception of schizophrenia and other thought disorders. In many cases the self-administration of drugs is actually the self-medication of symptoms associated with these coexisting psychiatric disorders. Healthcare professionals with anxiety-related symptoms often see the successful treatment of others with similar symptoms and may self-administer drugs with the same effects as those medications.

"I injured my back trying to grab a stack of films that was slipping to the ground and sustained multi-level disc bulges. At that time I was taking butalbital on most days and the neurologist prescribed tramadol for my pain. At the time, it wasn't really common knowledge that tramadol is addictive, but I'm sure many people were getting an inkling." By the spring of the year he was to graduate residency, Kramer realized that he was addicted to both drugs. "I attempted to stop the butalbital on my own. After three days I was hearing sitar music and there wasn't any band from New Delhi around—very frightening."

Kramer asked the neurologist for help withdrawing from the medication and he was admitted to the hospital. "The thing was, he admitted me to a general medicine floor but then didn't leave any orders for medicine or anything. I sat there the whole weekend going through withdrawal, with the sitar music getting louder, until I had a seizure." At that point, the medical resident must have figured out what was really going on and alerted the director of the radiology residency program. "I woke up and he was staring at me from a bedside chair. 'How long have you been planning this stunt?' was the first thing he said to me."

Kramer's program director was not the most empathetic of men. He knew perfectly well what was going on, but was willing to let it go as long as Kramer would be well enough to report for duty the following day. It seems the problem was not his addiction so much as his drug of choice. "In the Navy, captains and chiefs drink, but criminals take drugs." Admission to an addiction treatment center was not an option without a court marshal and a dishonorable discharge. "I would have probably had to do some time in the brig as well."

Kramer returned to work the next day. "I just started taking the butalbital again and the tramadol and began taking gabapentin and clonazepam as well. By the time part three of the board exam came around I was so miserable, addled, addicted and out of control that my poor performance was probably inevitable." Kramer failed the board exam but was working as a staff radiologist on one of the bases nonetheless. "I began drinking at night to try to get off the clonazepam, but I could never go more than three days without it. I woke up one morning on my bathroom floor. I had probably had another seizure. I didn't know what day it was and I hadn't even been drinking that day. I fell asleep on a watch and nobody could contact me for hours."

As a staff radiologist, Kramer's responsibilities included being immediately available to read emergency x-rays and other imaging studies on a timely basis. Patient management decisions were often based on his interpretation of these results, but he was in no condition to perform accurately. "I was lazy and I depended on a technician's interpretation more than I should have." On several occasions Kramer reported that patients had gallstones when they probably did not, misread one or two mammograms and missed an early stroke on a neuroradiology exam. "I realized that I hated my job. I couldn't stay awake, yet I couldn't be treated for prescription drug dependency." Kramer asked for and received a discharge from the Navy.

"I was discharged honorably, but they reported me to the National Practitioner Data Bank with a statement about me being hindered by prescription medication."

After that, things started to get worse. Having realized that radiology was no longer an option and not wanting to retrain in another medical specialty, Kramer opened an "aesthetic medicine" boutique practice. "I suppose because I was an addict I was also really interested in buprenorphine treatment for opioid addiction, so I got my certification and started treating people who wanted to look and feel better. I offered the whole medi-spa experience to anyone who was willing to pay. It was a cash business and we didn't take insurance. I started making a lot of money. Given my poor judgment, this was not a good combination." Still addicted to multiple prescription medications, Kramer now found himself with access to anything he wanted. "I didn't have to go to another physician to get what I needed; all I had to do was order it through the practice." Even though he could have any narcotic he wanted, Kramer still chose the medications which somehow made him feel like he thought he should. "All I wanted to do was make that underlying feeling of anxiety go away. Of all the things I could have, I took promethazine. I took it all the time; I just wanted to go to sleep."

As things continued to spiral out of control, Kramer began engaging in riskier behavior. "I became involved with one of my patients. She was a former heroin addict with chronic pain issues. I overreached my area of expertise and probably overprescribed, but I told myself that I had it under control. I never prescribed more than ten hydromorphone pills at a time, but this woman was at my office almost every day." As the two became enmeshed, boundaries began to blur and the patient, who had become at first a friend and then a lover, began to take a proprietary attitude. One of the women who was subleasing space in the medi-spa to perform facials "hadn't paid rent in a month or two and this woman went up to her and demanded that she pay." Shortly after that, the tenant notified the state medical board that something inappropriate was going on and an investigator from the Department of Consumer Affairs showed up at the spa. "I was home 'sick' and my manager called me at home and demanded that I come in and deal with this because she couldn't. I was a mess. I was getting high on anti-nausea medication and pain pills, my manager was apparently drinking alcohol at work and the facialist who reported me to the medical board was on methamphetamines!"

Not knowing what else to do, Kramer drank liquor heavily for the next several weeks. "I hid in my house while that damn investigator lurked around my gated community. It's possible he went home after the first few times I didn't answer the door, but I could swear he was still out there. Every time I peeked out the window I thought I saw him behind a bush or a car or standing by the mailbox." One evening, things got so bad Kramer decided he needed help. "I called my attorney, but he was just as drunk as I was."

Eventually the state medical board brought charges against Kramer. He lost everything. Because the investigation determined that he had not kept complete charts on all of the patients he had been prescribing controlled substances for, he was charged with gross negligence. The plea bargain his lawyer was able to arrange included mandated courses on ethics, professional boundaries, proper prescribing and record keeping. Because Kramer admitted to practicing while under the influence, he had to have an evaluation by an addiction medicine specialist and was ordered into treatment—ninety days at an inpatient facility. Kramer was allowed to keep his medical license but had to surrender his Drug Enforcement Agency license. The terms of the plea agreement stipulated that he could not work more than twenty-four hours in a week while on probation for the next seven years and that must be in a supervised setting with a practice monitor.

"I lost my home, because I couldn't pay the mortgage while in treatment. The ninety days of inpatient treatment cost me $30,000 and the monthly cost for the mandated support group and individual therapy, urine monitoring and administration fees is about $950. I'm pretty miserable and I'm at my rope's end financially. I spent every last cent of my savings, all of my belongings are in storage and my dog now lives with my parents. I'm quite sad and discouraged most of the time and deeply ashamed. I stay away from people, places and things that could be dangerous, but I also keep away from my healthy, professional friends as well, mostly out of shame."

Despite his insistence that he has no problem complying with the terms of his probation and that he has decided to "shut up and take direction" from his sponsor, it seems Kramer still harbors significant resentment about how much this whole process has cost him. "The court mandated that I have an evaluation by an addiction medicine specialist. Apparently there is only one in my area who is acceptable and I was charged $4,200," he said with bitterness. "My nursing colleagues in the program must suffer from a much less costly type of addiction, as they were evaluated for only $150."

Addiction is a disease of isolation and addicted healthcare professionals do not have the luxury of sharing their despair with anyone. Unlike what is commonly seen in the population of addicts who are not healthcare professionals, there is no "drug culture" in which addicts use together. Healthcare professionals who are addicted are alone and have much to lose if someone finds out what they are doing. It is rare that addicted healthcare professionals have confidants. If they are discovered, they fear they will lose their jobs, their licenses and the ability to secure other jobs as well as the respect of colleagues, family members and friends.

It is this fear of loss that prevents most addicted healthcare professionals from seeking treatment on their own. Ultimately, a fair number of these individuals will die, either from unintentional overdoses or by suicide. When formerly addicted healthcare professionals in recovery return to clinical work, it is important that colleagues and other personnel are supportive. They don't have to like it and they don't have to agree with the institutional policy which allows recovered professionals to return to work, but they need to understand that behaviors which encourage isolation can increase the risk for relapse and ultimately decrease patient safety.

Though different in many ways, Michelle and Kramer's stories are typical of addicted healthcare professionals. For most, there is a propensity toward addiction that begins as far back as early childhood. Often there is a history of excessive drinking and experimentation with other drugs of abuse prior to entering the healthcare field, but this is not always the case. There are many reasons why someone becomes addicted to prescription medications, but for most it is due to a predisposition coupled with exposure. In the next chapter, we will look at specific theories investigators have proposed to try to explain why someone would be predisposed to develop this disease in the first place. I believe that if we can understand who is at risk, we can develop strategies to intervene prior to exposure and prevent the harm to patients that often occurs.

CHAPTER 5

Why Some Healthcare Professionals Become Addicted

Physicians, nurses and other members of the healthcare team work in demanding, high-stress environments with ready access to large quantities of highly addictive drugs. Some find this tempting. Despite strict controls and accounting measures, drugs are relatively easy to divert for personal use.

Some people are able to use recreational drugs casually, while others become addicted quickly, suggesting that genetic susceptibility plays a role in the development of addiction and substance abuse. Individuals with novelty-seeking behavior traits may be both more likely to choose a particular medical specialty and more prone to develop addiction.

There is also an association between chemical dependence and other mental illnesses, such as depression or anxiety, that may contribute to the development of addiction in susceptible individuals. Exposure to trace quantities of highly addictive drugs used in the healthcare workplace may actually sensitize reward pathways by physically altering the structure of certain parts of the brain and promoting substance abuse. While none of these theories identifies a specific cause, they do suggest factors that may increase the risk of developing addictions among healthcare personnel.

Everybody's Job is Stressful, But Mine Is the Worst!

Mary, a nurse in recovery from addiction to oxycodone, currently works in a hospital in the Northeast. "The work is stressful; sometimes nursing can be a thankless job. We're expected to do too much for too many people in too short a time and when it doesn't get done or something bad happens then it's our fault. But if I couldn't handle it, I would have quit a long time ago." Mary injured her back on the job several years ago and required surgery. "The recovery was rough and I was the only one in the family with a job, so I had to go back to work. At first, the only way I could get out of bed was when I took the pills. When I took the oxycodone, it wasn't like I was high or goofy or anything; the pain just went away and I felt like I had the energy to do anything." Mary returned to work, still taking oxycodone. "The surgeon who fixed my back worked at the same hospital. He knew I was back at work. I couldn't keep going to him for the pain meds, so I started taking them from the hospital supply."

When Mary was first prescribed oxycodone, it was to meet a valid medical need. She continued to take the drug out of what was, in her mind, necessity, so that she could continue working to support her family. Her story is not uncommon. "Nurses are paid a lot for what they do. Often they make more than their spouses and most of the time the spouse who makes less is the man. That can really change the dynamic in a traditional marriage; you have to have a really strong relationship to make that work. I can see how that kind of stress would drive you to drink—my husband did—but I never felt like the stress of the job itself contributed to my using." Mary's diversion was discovered when the pharmacist crosschecked the dispensing records with the physicians' orders. "I was immediately fired, no questions asked. They reported me to the state board of nursing and I lost my license. It took me two years to get it back. Now *that* was stressful."

The overwhelming majority of healthcare professionals who are not addicted cite stress and the availability of drugs as the main reasons why one of their colleagues would choose to abuse the medications intended for patients and then become addicted to them. But almost all healthcare professionals work in highly stressful positions and most of these people do not end up using these medications on themselves. Stress is a concept that is difficult to define and its effect on the development of addiction in persons at risk is not clear. When one asks addicted healthcare professionals what they think contributed to the development of their addictions, the stress of the job is rarely cited as the primary cause. All professions come with their own sets of unique stressors and people who choose to work in these kinds of high-stress environments may actually thrive under this type of pressure. It may be, then, that it is not the actual presence of stress that is causative, but rather healthcare professionals' unhealthy responses to stress that are the harbinger of substance abuse and eventual addiction.

Michelle, the nurse in recovery whose story was told earlier, began taking pills while working as a pharmacy technician during nursing school. She thinks that stress is definitely a contributing factor but also thinks that people who are attracted to stress and drama may be attracted to drugs and alcohol as well. "It goes with the personality type. Some people thrive in stressful environments; we need the constant stimulation. We function well under pressure, so it isn't the stress that drives us to use drugs or to drink to excess. It's just an association." The need for stimulation is satisfied for some by work-related stress, but it can also be satisfied through the use of drugs and alcohol.

There are others, however, who cite the stress associated with the high demands of being a healthcare professional as directly influencing their decisions to abuse drugs. Willie Ames is a nursing instructor at a community college. "I've been a nurse for decades and I've worked at the bedside most of the time." Initially he started abusing by drinking alcohol to excess. "I drank to relieve stress at the end of the long twelve-hour shifts in hospital nursing." Willie believes that the high-stress environment in which healthcare professionals work is definitely a contributing factor to the development of his addiction. "That is what encouraged me to drink." Willie added hydrocodone, a prescription narcotic medication similar to codeine, when he was prescribed the pills for postoperative pain after gallbladder surgery. He continued to drink as well as take narcotics.

As the way in which healthcare is delivered in the United States changes, it is likely that the demands on healthcare professionals will only increase. Most facilities are already operating at close to maximum capacity, with doctors working between seventy and ninety hours a week and nurses working long shifts, often with mandatory overtime. These professionals must consistently perform at extremely high levels, internalize their emotions and be able to make life or death decisions in real time. Making a comparison between baseball and the practice of medicine, Mark, a gastroenterologist, said: "What's a good average? .300? What does that really mean anyway? That this guy who's supposed to be one of the best players in the game only gets on base 30 percent of the time. Can you imagine if I got the diagnosis right only 30 percent of the time? And we pay these athletes how much for this performance? We're expected to be right 100 percent of the time and in this new system, if we're wrong we don't get paid!" Healthcare professionals work in very demanding and emotionally taxing environments.

The level of expectations and stress on healthcare professionals will only increase as we adopt the changes associated with healthcare reform. If we are not careful to allow time for decompression and build safety nets into this new system, it is possible that we may start to see job stress and frustration cited more often as the reason why healthcare professionals choose to abuse drugs.

Genetics: Sometimes Blaming Your Parents Makes Sense

The disease of alcoholism was formally recognized by the American Medical Association in 1956, paving the way for medically based treatments and, perhaps more importantly, the coverage of these treatments by some health insurance plans.[1] Access to adequate treatment for addictive disorders has always been limited, primarily by restricted access to financial resources, but the recognition of addiction to any drug of abuse as a disease in 1987 increased access to treatment through extended insurance coverage.

The designation of addiction as a disease and not a failure of moral fortitude prompted inquiries into the causes of addictive disorders. Considerable research has been done involving the development of addiction in persons at risk that suggests a genetic component.[2] Studies that look retrospectively at genetically identical twins separated at birth and raised in different environments suggest that about 40 percent of the risk that an individual will develop an addiction is related to genetics and the other 60 percent is related to environmental factors.[3]

Have you ever taken drugs? Have you ever drunk alcohol? How did these substances make you feel? The drug-taking experience is a highly subjective one. Just as there are genes which determine the color of your eyes and hair, there are genes which determine how you will respond to alcohol and other psychoactive drugs. Most people under the influence of alcohol or other drugs will have the same signs and symptoms, which suggest to the casual observer that they are intoxicated. Many of us have seen a person at a party or a ballgame who has had too much to drink: his speech is slurred, his gait unsteady. These are common and expected effects of alcohol, but just like one person may be a "happy drunk" and another may become quite surly, the interpretation of these effects by the user is altered by their prior experiences, coexisting psychiatric disorders or character traits and genetics. Take, for example, two friends smoking marijuana together. They both share the same marijuana cigarette and both exhibit the same outward signs of intoxication: decreased blood pressure due to relaxation of the blood vessels and increased heart rate due to stimulation of the sympathetic nervous system. Yet these two friends experience these symptoms differently. They both report heightened sensory perception and a distortion of space and time, but while one interprets these feelings as euphoric, the other finds these sensations are anxiety-provoking and reports feelings of dysphoria. Two people taking the same drug can have very different experiences and these differences are to some degree related to genetics.

Specific genetic factors have been identified which may account for the subjective differences between users of the same drug as well as the predilection for the development of addiction.[4] For a drug to have psychoactive properties, it must contain an element that, when introduced to the body, is able to enter the brain of the user, bind to an existing receptor and make a change in the brain's chemistry. In the case of marijuana, this element is tetrahydrocannabinol (THC) and the receptor in the brain it binds to is the cannabinoid receptor. Activation of the cannabinoid receptor by THC changes the relative levels of different brain chemicals, which gives the user the feelings associated with getting high on marijuana.

While the two friends in our example both have cannabinoid receptors to which THC can bind, the gene that produces this receptor is different in each person so the drug produces a different response to the same drug. Maybe one receptor allows the drug to bind more tightly; possibly the receptor produces an exaggerated response; perhaps the response invoked by binding to the drug is altogether different. We don't understand exactly how this works, but in the friend who experiences marijuana intoxication as euphoric, activation of his cannabinoid receptor probably results in an increase of dopamine, which makes a person feel really good. In the friend who experiences the same drug as dysphoria, activation of his cannabinoid receptor might result in a decrease of dopamine. This change in the relative levels of different brain chemicals is involved with the reinforcement of drug seeking behaviors associated with drugs of abuse.

Now we will apply this example to two healthcare professionals who have the opportunity to experience intoxication with a drug such as fentanyl. Ignoring for the moment the factors which would lead to the individuals' choosing to self-administer the drug in the first place, their individual responses will depend to some extent on the structure of the fentanyl receptors in their brains, which in turn depend on the genes that they carry. One healthcare worker may have genes that produce receptors that are hypersensitive to narcotics while the other may have receptors that invoke a less exaggerated response.

The same dose of the same drug will invoke a markedly different response in these two genetically different individuals. Reinforcement of drug-using behavior occurs more readily in individuals with hypersensitive receptors and responds to much lower doses. This exaggerated response to lower levels of the drug increases the likelihood that dependence will develop. Chronic use results in the development of tolerance and sensitization, which further reinforces drug using behavior and at much smaller doses in individuals who are genetically susceptible.

Alcohol abuse is the most common form of substance abuse in our society and many families can point to multiple generations with affected individuals. Many healthcare professionals in recovery can identify a strong family history of alcoholism in multiple generations, even if alcohol was not their personal drug of choice. Karen is a certified nurse-midwife who has not been practicing clinically for almost a decade due to ongoing issues with her addiction to prescription medications. Though she does not report having any issues with alcohol herself, she does have a strong family history. "My dad was an alcoholic who was 'saved' and became a minister when I was two years old. He had one cousin who died of alcoholism, another cousin, who was a sibling to the first one, who had a problem with drugs and was also an alcoholic and recently committed suicide, and an uncle who died of alcoholism." Chuck is another healthcare professional in recovery with a strong family history. "My father, my grandfather and many other relatives all died of alcohol-related diseases. I was too young to understand what they were talking about at the time, but I remember hearing about my father's brother, whom they said always 'needed his dope,' so I guess there's a family history of drug abuse too."

Substance abuse and addiction are prevalent within multiple generations of some families, so it makes sense that there should be an associated genetic component. In fact, a strong family history of drug or alcohol abuse is the strongest predictor of drug or alcohol abuse in healthcare professionals. This genetic predisposition, however, is just that: a predisposition. There are many factors that contribute to the development of substance use disorders in predisposed individuals. This genetic susceptibility probably plays a role in the transition from substance use to dependence and from chronic use to addiction.

Personality Traits

Drugs of abuse activate the reward system in the brain and reinforce drug using behavior. We know that these changes in behavior are reflective of physical changes in the physiology and chemistry of the brain. Most individuals who experiment with drugs of abuse do not become addicted or physically dependent on them, but there is a subset of individuals who do.[5] What makes these people different from people who can casually use drugs and not become dependent on them? Is this more a reflection of the personality type of an individual or does it depend on the properties of the drug itself? Are healthcare professionals more at risk for addiction because the personality traits that make them more effective members of the healthcare team also make them more likely to develop addiction?

Despite considerable research into the topic, we have yet to discover the presence of an "addictive personality," someone who is at high risk for developing the disease of addiction because of personality traits. There are common personality stereotypes which persist, because to some extent they hold an element of truth and consistency. Not all surgeons are obstinate and conceited, but enough are that one can say an individual is behaving like a surgeon and most healthcare professionals know what is meant. Leslie has been managing the operating room schedule at the anesthesia control desk of a large teaching hospital for decades. "Do you know what the difference between God and a surgeon is?" he asks. "God don't think he's a surgeon." It is more likely that certain personality traits play a role in the development and progression of the disease, even if they are not causative in nature.

Greg, a rheumatologist from the Midwest who likes extreme sports, has struggled with addiction to hydrocodone for the past ten years. "It started when I was injured in a climbing accident many years ago. I was with a team trying to make an ascent to the Everest summit. We were only a day out of base camp when I slipped and fractured my leg. It wasn't anything dramatic or sensational like what happened later that year when two people died, but it hurt like hell. I had to be carried back to base camp and it took forever to get to a hospital. By the time I got back to the United States, the bones had somewhat healed and had to be re-broken and set properly. The rehabilitation was a long, painful process and I had to take a lot of narcotics just to be able to get around. The funny thing was, I actually felt more awake when I was taking them, like I had more energy and the motivation to do great things. I wasn't slow or sedated or anything like what I would have expected."

Greg's experience is not uncommon and many people who become addicted to narcotics report experiencing a paradoxical reaction to these drugs. Since we know that each individual metabolizes narcotics and other medications at different rates, it makes sense that there will be some people who respond quite differently to the same medications. As I listened to him recount his adventures, it occurred to me that Greg also has red hair, a trait which itself does not confer on him an altered level of drug metabolism, but is thought to be located in close enough proximity to a gene that does, as many redheaded individuals share an increased tolerance of all types of medications.

"I've always been someone who likes to take risks," Greg continued. "Extreme sports like mountain climbing, river rafting, skydiving. You name it and I've done it and if I haven't, I want to." Rheumatology seems like an odd field for someone with such a proclivity for adventure, but it seems that Greg's medical practice was only a means to an end. "I chose rheumatology because the hours are reasonable, the pay is decent and, if I want to take six weeks off to climb Mount Everest, I can. When I got back to work after I broke my leg and realized I wouldn't be able to do any extreme sports for a while, I got really bored. I started taking hydrocodone from the office and found that things were much more interesting if I was high. I thought I was much more productive and I certainly enjoyed my work much more, so I was in a good mood, but eventually I was caught. The office manager told my partners that I had been dipping into the practice's supplies and they sent me to rehab."

Greg completed an inpatient program designed for addicted healthcare professionals and was allowed to return to clinical practice provided he participate in a five-year monitoring program. "They assigned one of my partners to be my practice monitor and a gastroenterologist who works in the same building agreed to be my urine monitor." The state in which Greg was licensed to practice medicine required participants in the monitoring program to submit urine samples on a regular basis for analysis. "It's supposed to be random, but this guy was doing me a favor and it was easier for him if I came by his office once a week on Fridays. I knew I could use drugs on the weekends and I would still drop a clean urine by the end of the week, but I chose not to use."

That is, until Greg's risk-taking behavior resulted in another injury requiring treatment with narcotics. "I was making a bonfire for my kids. I poured gasoline over a giant pile of wood and when I lit it the whole thing exploded. I was covered with burns. Over 50 percent of my body had second and third degree burns. I don't know if you know anything about burn injuries, but they hurt like hell. I was in the hospital for eight weeks and when I came home I was hooked on pills again. I started writing prescriptions for hydrocodone in my patients' names and filling them myself." Eventually the pharmacist became suspicious and Greg once again entered an inpatient rehabilitation program.

Healthcare professionals are, by nature, driven to maintain extremely high standards. The perfectionists among them rise to the top of what is a very elite group to begin with and it is not surprising to note that addicted medical students and residents in treatment are often in the top 20 percent of their classes. Healthcare professionals who enter treatment later in life are often high performing in their careers prior to developing addiction. The diagnosis of compulsive personality disorder or the presence of these traits is very common in this population and likely explains why these people are highly functioning to begin with, although since these traits are likely helpful for any healthcare professional to have, it is possible that many who do not develop addiction and require treatment also share these personality traits.

An Addicted Psychiatrist with an Anxiety Disorder

Amy, a psychiatrist with a private practice, recounted her experience with addiction to prescription medications. "I've always been a little high-strung. I'm nervous to begin with, but when something goes wrong or I'm under a lot of pressure I get really anxious." Amy was a very shy child and spent a lot of time by herself when she was growing up. She had few close friends and often did not relate well to others in her peer group. "I think my parents actually suspected I was autistic at one point." Though she never was formally diagnosed with an anxiety disorder, Amy always felt that her experiences were not the same as everyone else's. "In high school everyone else seemed to have it all together. I was a mess." Unable to quiet her nerves enough to deal with everyday life, Amy threw herself into her studies. "I worked hard in high school mostly because I didn't have anything else to do. I got into a good college and went directly into medical school. It wasn't until then that I was able to diagnose myself."

Amy's experience as a healthcare professional with an undiagnosed mental illness is typical.[6] She knew something was wrong, but it wasn't until she was in medical school that she was able to figure out what it was. "When I was in medical school, my father became critically ill and I ended up in the emergency room thinking I was having a heart attack. I was having palpitations and was convinced my heart was racing because I was going to die. After I had the full workup, blood tests, EKG, even an echocardiogram, they referred me to a psychiatrist. He diagnosed me with an anxiety disorder and prescribed alprazolam. He also gave me a medication so my heart wouldn't race. The alprazolam was really supposed to be for when things got really bad, but as far as I was concerned, things were always really bad, so I took it every day. I was so stoned I don't even really remember my dad's funeral."

Amy continued to take the alprazolam throughout medical school, getting her prescription filled at first from the psychiatrist who prescribed them and then, after he refused to refill her prescription, from the attending physicians on her various clinical rotations. "Self-medicating is so easy when you know what symptoms you're treating. As physicians, we know what these drugs do and which ones to take to make the anxiety go away, but covering up the problem by treating the symptoms and not the cause doesn't make things better." Eventually it became clear to most people around her that she had a problem and during her residency in psychiatry Amy was sent to a treatment program for addicted medical professionals. "I was taking so much alprazolam that I couldn't function. The anxiety was gone, but there was nothing left. It was as if I had become dead inside; I was numb to the world."

Speaking to me several years after undergoing detoxification and completing treatment at an inpatient facility, Amy seemed very calm and composed. "The anxiety is still there and it's a lot better, but sometimes I still feel like a duck." An odd look from me prompted further explanation: "You know how a duck looks all calm above the water but meanwhile her legs are frantically paddling just below the surface?" It's a fitting analogy, but I inquired what it must be like to have to live with the constant agitation. "I had to learn how to deal with the anxiety in a more constructive and positive way," she explained. "Instead of trying to make it go away with medications, I try to use it to my advantage." Amy now heads the mental health program at a medical school. "I see a lot of students going through the same things I did and it's wonderful to be in a position to help." I have to ask, but the answer is clear: "I don't prescribe them alprazolam."

Coexisting Psychopathy

When we consider the association between chemical dependence and another mental illness, it is often difficult to know which came first. In addicted individuals, it is impossible to diagnose a psychiatric disorder, as many of the signs and symptoms of these disorders can also be attributed to intoxication or withdrawal. While individuals under evaluation or in treatment for substance abuse should have an evaluation with subsequent management of any psychiatric conditions, drug-dependent individuals must be clean for a period of time before any signs, symptoms or behaviors can be attributed to mental illness alone.

Jin used to work as a pharmacy technician before he lost his job because of his diversion of prescription narcotics. "I was miserable. I mean really miserable; so miserable that everyone around me was also miserable. I started taking oxycodone from work, because I had heard on the news that people were using it to get high and I wanted to try it. I had heard in the story about how people crushed the pills and snorted it to get around the time released formula, so that's how I took it. The high was amazing, like nothing I'd ever felt before. I didn't want to do anything else and if I couldn't get any I was really depressed. My girlfriend knew something wasn't right, but I just told her I was feeling depressed. The thing was, I wasn't lying; I really was depressed. She made me go to see a shrink and he gave me an antidepressant, but that didn't make me any better so they also gave me a mood stabilizer."

In fact, the combination of medications Jin was taking and the high dose of oxycodone he was using had the opposite effect. "One evening I just lost it. She said something to me that set me off and I threatened to kill her and our son. She left that night and took our boy with her. After she was gone, I took every pill I could find. I was so far gone I didn't know what to do. I didn't really want to die, but I couldn't keep going on like this." If his girlfriend hadn't called the police, Jin would probably have died that night. "They found me unconscious and took me to the emergency room." Jin had reached the point where he had become sick and tired of being sick and tired. "The ER doc sent me to this place where they have meetings for people with addictions. It's like alcoholics anonymous but for people who have problems with drugs."

Karen, the certified nurse-midwife whom we discussed earlier, was diagnosed with bipolar disorder six months into "white knuckle" sobriety, but she was diagnosed only after she had been sober for a sufficient period of time. "In retrospect, a lot of the symptoms I was having were probably due to my psychiatric illness and I was self-medicating." Her treatment for addiction included abstinence from any mood-altering drugs, but after six months sober she still had persistent symptoms suggestive of psychiatric illness. Now on oxcarbazepine and bupropion, many of the feelings that used to compel her to use drugs are gone. "I take trazadone sometimes to sleep and topiramate to control weight gain as an adjunct to therapy, but the meds make it a lot easier to remain sober."

Healthcare professionals are not immune to the long-term effects of emotional or physical trauma and post-traumatic stress disorder (PTSD) plays a significant role in the development of addiction to alcohol and other drugs. Exposure to combat increases the risk of addiction in soldiers, so it makes sense that exposure to the physical and emotional trauma of war would have a similar effect on the healthcare professionals tasked with treating war injuries. But the physicians, nurses and other healthcare professionals who work in emergency departments, trauma centers or war zones during active conflict may not be the only ones at risk for developing PTSD and subsequent addiction.

A different kind of trauma, the trauma of childhood sexual abuse, has been associated with the development of propofol abuse. Most healthcare professionals who abuse propofol are anesthesiologists, presumably because of easy access to this drug and familiarity with its properties, but they also share other characteristics.[7]

The majority of people who abuse propofol are women and most report suffering trauma during childhood, often of a sexual nature. These people are often unable to sleep and they describe a desire to block out the world. It is this common history of psychological or physical trauma, such as rape or childhood sexual abuse, which may help explain the drug's appeal. When given in low doses, propofol creates a dissociative state which some describe as an "out-of-body" experience. For some, it provides a much-needed escape from reality. Many who begin to abuse propofol do so to relieve insomnia and to overcome the hyperarousal that is common in people with PTSD. The strength of the connection between the development of propofol abuse and a history of childhood trauma is greater than that which is seen with any other drug, including alcohol. It is likely that, as access to this drug moves beyond the healthcare setting, more civilians will begin to enter treatment specifically for addiction to propofol.

Workplace Exposure

When one examines the class of drugs abused by different types of healthcare professionals it becomes clear that addicted healthcare workers tend to self-administer the drugs that they are comfortable with; that is, those drugs that they administer to others on a regular basis.[8] This explains the observation that anesthesia care providers abuse narcotics more frequently than any other class of drug and those involved with the psychiatric field more commonly abuse benzodiazepines. Emergency medicine personnel frequently encounter patients under the influence of street drugs and perhaps because of this they are more likely to abuse drugs such as cocaine and marijuana. While existing data illustrate these trends, this is by no means a set rule. Healthcare professionals in any field can become addicted to any drug.[9]

The increased risk of addiction in anesthesia care providers presents a special case of workplace exposure. Not only do these healthcare professionals have ready access to highly addictive narcotics such as fentanyl, but also they are regularly exposed to measurable levels of these agents present in the exhaled breath of patients receiving them. Low doses of these drugs have been shown to induce physical changes in the brain. It is possible that exposure to even minute quantities of these drugs through passive administration, such as by breathing in what someone else has just exhaled, could sensitize the reward pathways in the brain and reinforce drug-using behavior.[10] Narcotics are known to alter the brain's chemistry, typically by changing the relative levels of the neurotransmitters gamma-aminobutyric acid (GABA), dopamine and serotonin, so that drug-seeking behavior is favored over the rational evaluation of the risks of such actions. Anesthesia care providers who become sensitized through exposure in the workplace are at even greater risk for dependence and addiction and may actually develop withdrawal if they are away from work for more than a day.[11] Theoretically, these individuals, recognizing the symptoms of withdrawal for what they are, could use narcotics to alleviate the withdrawal they feel when away from the exposure.

Workplace exposure is not limited to anesthesia care providers in the operating room and can also include exposure through access to drugs. Some physicians develop addiction to prescription drugs like oxycodone and alprazolam early in their careers, shortly after obtaining a medical license and a prescription pad. It is likely that these individuals abused other drugs or alcohol previously and the newfound access to controlled drugs is too much temptation to resist. As new narcotics and other medications with abuse potential are brought to market, pharmaceutical company representatives encourage healthcare professionals to prescribe their new products. Samples of these drugs are often provided and can easily be taken home for personal use by anyone with access to the cabinets where they are stored. Changes in the types of drugs abused by healthcare professionals as reported by treatment centers often parallel the development of new drugs and, more importantly, portend the development of abuse of these drugs in the civilian population. Just as the increasing frequency of tramadol abuse in the population of healthcare professionals treated for addiction in the late 1990s was a harbinger for abuse in the general population, the increased incidence of misuse of certain drugs by healthcare professionals should serve as a warning to the DEA that these drugs have significant abuse potential and should be controlled.

To people who have no personal experience with drug abuse, it may seem perplexing why others choose to behave in such self-destructive manners. This can be even more troubling when the addict is a highly motivated medical professional who has invested multiple years in education and training, yet seems to be unable to stop using. For the friends and family members of addicted healthcare professionals, having a better understanding of the multiple reasons why these people may be at increased risk for developing addiction may or may not make it easier to accept. Perhaps the realization that these behaviors do not represent a choice so much as a reflection of an underlying brain disease will make it easier to cope with.

In this chapter we have discussed a number of the more popular and plausible theories proposed to explain why this troubling observation is accurate. What is perhaps more striking than the large number of healthcare professionals who become addicted to prescription medications each year is the even higher number of people who do not. Given the easy access to highly addictive agents and the character traits which so many in the healthcare professions share, one might expect to find a greater number of individuals addicted to prescription drugs. This is an intriguing situation and hopefully future research will be able to identify either genes or other characteristics that are protective against developing addiction, even with exposure.

CHAPTER 6

What Types of Prescription Drugs Healthcare Professionals Abuse

Addicted healthcare professionals have ready access to pretty much any drug they desire. Want to stay up late? There's a drug for that. Been up too long and need to come down? There's another one for that. These drugs are marketed to the general public through powerful advertising campaigns that urge patients to "ask your doctor" if a particular drug is right for them or not. Often these medications have significant abuse potential which may be unappreciated by both the physicians prescribing them as well as the patients who are asking for them. We have become a society that expects immediate solutions to every problem and drugs hold the promise of a quick fix: "Just take one of these and everything will be alright." As the demand to increase productivity, to decrease costs and to preserve patient safety marches forward, it is only human nature to look for shortcuts. Many healthcare professionals who become addicted to prescription medications report that they initially began using these drugs not as an escape from the pressures of life and work, but as a means to become more fully involved and productive.

Michael Jackson's Drug of Choice

Michael Jackson liked propofol. He liked it a lot and it ended up being the death of him, but many people who abuse this drug are not patients but rather their healthcare professionals. Propofol is a medication used to induce general anesthesia that most people who do not work in the healthcare field had never heard of before the tragic death of pop culture icon Michael Jackson during the summer of 2009.

Propofol must be administered intravenously to work, so the addict needs to have access to the equipment necessary to inject or infuse it. The drug works quickly; so quickly, in fact, that within seconds after the injection the user begins to lose consciousness. By the time the medication has traveled from the injection site to the brain, the user is entering a state of general anesthesia. Depending on the amount of propofol injected, the user will either begin to wake up in five to ten minutes or stop breathing and die. There is a very narrow range between the dose that will produce the desired effects of unconsciousness or semi-consciousness and the dose that will stop the user from breathing on his or her own.

When this drug is used in clinical practice the patient is always supervised by an anesthesia care provider, who is trained in airway support and cardiopulmonary resuscitation to assist the patient if he or she does require help with breathing. Despite the intimate knowledge of how this medication works that most healthcare professionals with access to this drug have, there are many factors that can alter the effectiveness of the drug and miscalculations resulting in overdose when self-administered are common.

Propofol is a short-acting agent that has few residual effects. Addicts who abuse this drug report waking up with a general sense of well-being, feeling well-rested. Because of this, regular abuse has been called "pro-napping" and is common among addicted healthcare professionals who work long and stressful shifts. With little time for restorative sleep, it may seem that a "pro-nap" can provide a much-needed break, but unconsciousness is not sleep and these "naps" do not provide the restoration that actual sleep does.

Addicts report a number of different feelings after propofol administration, ranging from a mild feeling of well-being to that of elation, euphoria and sexual disinhibition. The drug consistently scores high on the likability scales that medical researchers use and most experts who study the addictive properties of drugs consider it to have significant abuse potential.

Propofol is not a drug that lends itself to safe self-administration. Rick, an anesthesiologist, became addicted to propofol as a resident physician. "I initially tried propofol during my first year as an anesthesia resident. We kept it in the anesthesia cart with all the other medications that weren't controlled. Anyone who had access to the cart could take it and no one would ever know." People who have access to these carts include not only members of the anesthesia care team (medical doctors, certified registered nurse anesthetists, anesthesiologist assistants and anesthesia residents), but also the medical students rotating through anesthesia or surgery clerkships, members of the surgical team (surgeons and their assistants, surgical residents, scrub technicians and surgical nurses), the anesthesia technicians who stock the carts and even members of the janitorial staff who clean and turn over the room between cases and at the end of the day. "Unlike fentanyl or morphine, which I had to check out from the pharmacy and account for at the end of the day, nobody ever knew how much propofol was in these carts at any given time. I took a couple bottles and the equipment I needed to inject it home with me and nobody even missed it."

The first time Rick injected himself with propofol, he was alone. The drug worked so quickly that Rick was unconscious before he had finished injecting the contents of the syringe. "I woke up on the floor, flat on my face. There was blood everywhere. I had a bloody nose and the IV I had placed in my arm had become disconnected, so blood was leaking out of that as well. I could have very easily died, but I didn't, and when I woke up I felt great. I loved the oblivion; I couldn't get enough." Soon Rick started injecting himself at work. "I put a catheter in place so I could repeatedly inject myself throughout the day. At first I did it when I was on a break in the call room, but it wasn't long before I did it while I was in the operating room." Eventually, a dose miscalculation resulted in an overdose during a case while he was supposed to be taking care of a patient. "I took a face dive in the operating room. Just slid forward off my chair and wound up flat on the floor in the middle of a case."

Once discovered, Rick was removed from clinical practice and sent to an inpatient treatment facility that specializes in the treatment of addicted healthcare professionals. Fortunately, neither Rick nor his patient was injured during this episode, but not everyone has been so lucky. Many individuals who become addicted to propofol end up overdosing and dying alone.

Because it only lasts for a short period of time, the volume of propofol required to maintain regular use would be difficult to obtain without being detected if it were a controlled substance. Despite ample evidence that it has significant abuse potential, propofol is still not tightly controlled by the Drug Enforcement Administration (DEA). It remains readily available to healthcare professionals who practice in areas where it is used and it is likely that access to this powerful and potentially dangerous drug with high addiction potential is responsible for a number of deaths.

New to the market is fos-propofol, a prodrug formulation of propofol originally intended to have all of the good qualities of propofol but not the bad ones. As a prodrug, it has to be metabolized to propofol in the body before it becomes active. Because of this, fos-propofol has a significantly longer onset of action than propofol (four minutes versus thirty seconds), but once metabolized its clinical profile is the same. The manufacturers of fos-propofol worked hard to design an agent with the same clinical profile as propofol but without the sometimes harmful side effects. Unfortunately, this new drug shares the same abuse potential that propofol does. Recognizing this, the DEA has classified fos-propofol as a schedule IV drug, indicating that it shares the same abuse potential as drugs like diazepam, alprazolam and zolpidem. (Under the comprehensive Drug Abuse Prevention and Control Act of 1970, the DEA classifies controlled substances into five schedules based on potential for abuse, accepted medical use and safety under medical supervision.) Though fos-propofol has not been on the market long enough to know accurately how people are currently abusing it, it is likely that reports will soon begin to surface. What is more disturbing, however, is that propofol remains unscheduled and not controlled by the DEA.

Increasing Danger

Although any prescription medication can be misused, drugs from these three classes are most commonly abused: narcotics, which are usually prescribed to treat pain, central nervous system (CNS) depressants, which are used to treat anxiety and sleep disorders, and stimulants, which are commonly prescribed to treat attention deficit/hyperactivity disorder (ADHD) and narcolepsy. Even though generally there is not an increased prevalence of drug abuse and addiction among healthcare providers as compared to the general population, when one looks more closely at the data there is a difference in the rates of addiction to specific types of drugs. The types of drugs abused by healthcare professionals do not necessarily reflect the rates of addiction to these drugs in the local or regional population in which they practice but rather more closely reflect the rates of addiction to these types of drugs by provider types regardless of location. It makes sense intuitively that if a person is going to use drugs, he or she is more likely to choose the ones he or she has access to. That's what we see when we look at the different kinds of drugs that different types of healthcare providers are abusing.

Narcotics are analgesic, pain-relieving medications with a wide range of uses. Oral medications such as hydrocodone, propoxyphene, hydromorphone, meperidine, oxycodone and codeine may be prescribed for chronic pain or for use for a limited period of time, such as during a postoperative period. Medications available in injectable forms, such as morphine, fentanyl or sufentanil, are often used to alleviate severe pain associated with surgery. All of these narcotic medications have effective pain-relieving properties but also produce intense euphoria and carry a high risk of addiction and physical dependence if misused.

Narcotic medications effectively change the way a person experiences pain. By attaching to specific proteins called opioid receptors, which are found in the brain and spinal cord, these medications trigger the release of brain chemicals that either lessen the intensity of the pain perceived by the user or eliminate it entirely. One patient described the odd sensation of being aware of the pain but no longer experiencing it as pain: "It was as if the morphine had come between me and the pain. I was still aware of its existence, but it was somehow disconnected from me. I could feel the pain, but it didn't hurt. Instead, I felt quite pleasant."

Because of these properties, narcotic medications are often used in the treatment of a wide variety of medical problems that create pain or discomfort in the patient. In addition to their role in treating or preventing pain, narcotic medications also affect regions of the brain that mediate what one perceives as pleasure. Another patient described the experience of receiving hydromorphone as one of the most pleasurable experiences of his life: "The headache was unbearable. I felt as though I would die if the pain were to continue for much longer, but then in an instant it was gone, replaced almost immediately by a feeling of warmth and pleasure and well-being the likes of which I had never experienced before. As the smile grew across my face the nurse who had just given me the [hydromorphone] gave me a knowing glance, as if we were suddenly coconspirators in some private affair."

The initial euphoria or sense of well-being that many narcotics produce is a common reason why many people repeatedly abuse these medications. As these people soon find out, subsequent experiences are never as good as the first time. Anyone who wears glasses has had a similar experience. The first time you put the glasses on the world is suddenly clear, everything comes into focus and you see things that you never saw before. Things are never as clear as that again and it's the same with the first experience with any of these addictive drugs of abuse.

Anesthesia care providers, the group of healthcare professionals who provide anesthesia services for surgery or painful procedures, include anesthesiologists (physicians trained in the administration of anesthesia), certified registered nurse anesthetists (registered nurses with supplemental training in providing anesthesia) and anesthesiologist assistants (physician assistants with specific training in the administration of anesthesia). These people represent a diverse group with varying degrees of education and training who all work in the same field and have access to some of the most addictive medications. Fentanyl, a synthetic morphine-like narcotic medication used in almost every anesthetic administered today, is 100 times more potent than heroin and contains no impurities (currently available clandestinely manufactured heroin only contains 30 to 60 percent heroin, depending on the source).[1]

In 2006, someone was able to produce pharmaceutical grade fentanyl in a secret laboratory somewhere south of Chicago.[2] The intent was to use the fentanyl to increase the potency of heroin so that the heroin could be further cut with impurities, increasing the profit for the distributors. Apparently it is much less expensive to produce fentanyl domestically than it is to import heroin. In fact, 250 micrograms of fentanyl purchased in bulk from a supplier costs only twenty-seven cents and most of that cost is for the glass ampule that it comes in, but one needs a DEA license to purchase it. In this case, the distributor didn't understand how powerful this medication was and soon heroin addicts in the Chicago area were dying. That summer, some of the fentanyl-laced heroin made it to New York and addicts started dying there too. Since dealers of street drugs depend on repeat sales, these distributors abandoned the idea, for the moment anyway.

Anesthesia care providers have unique access to fentanyl and other so-called "major narcotics" with high potency and addictive potential, so it is no surprise that when one of these people ends up entering a drug treatment facility, 60 to 75 percent of the time it is for addiction to one of these agents.[3]

CNS depressants such as tranquilizers or sedatives like diazepam, alprazolam and estazolam, commonly prescribed to treat anxiety, acute stress reactions, panic attacks, convulsions and sleep disorders, slow normal brain function and increase reaction time. In higher doses, some of these medications can be used as premedication prior to general anesthesia or as general anesthetics themselves. Barbiturates, such as methohexital, thiopental, mephobarbital and sodium pentobarbital, are used as preanesthetics, promoting sleep.

If you're wondering how dangerous some of these medications can be, consider this: Thiopental is the choice drug used for the lethal injection method of execution. It is no longer available in the United States, because it is now manufactured only in Italy and the Italian government will not allow this medication to be exported to the United States knowing it will be used for this purpose. CNS depressants are usually prescribed only for short-term problems because of the quick development of tolerance and risk of addiction. Some newer medications such as zolpidem, zaleplon and eszopiclone are now more commonly prescribed to treat sleep disorders. Despite their classification as non-benzodiazepines that act at a subset of the benzodiazepine receptors, they still have a significant risk for abuse and addiction and are often used as substitute drugs when narcotics or other benzodiazepines are not available. Since psychiatrists have more experience with prescribing these medications than any other group of healthcare professionals, it is not surprising that the drug of choice for these individuals entering treatment is most commonly a CNS depressant.

It's not just injectable drugs like fentanyl and propofol that healthcare professionals have access to; the majority of prescription medications that are diverted for illicit uses each year are in tablet or pill form. Though at times it may seem like it, members of the anesthesia care team do not have a monopoly on the abuse of prescription narcotics.

Charles, formerly medical director of a family practice clinic, a well-respected physician and businessman in a small Southern town, had an addiction to prescription medications. "I started using prescription drugs when I was thirty-eight years old, about ten years into practice." Despite his considerable education, training and experience, the only job he has been able to get recently is entirely unrelated to medicine. With nowhere to go after completing the year of outpatient treatment for his addiction, he chose to stay as an employee at the sober living facility where he was housed during his first year of recovery. As compensation for his work as the resident manager, Charles does not have to pay rent and receives a meager weekly stipend.

Charles reported prior alcohol abuse but denied that it was ever an issue. "I drank in college but never to excess or to a greater extent than what other people around me were doing. If everyone at the party was getting drunk, then I got drunk, but only on weekends or during social activities. I never drank during the week." Charles started using prescriptions because they were readily available. "We had samples of hydrocodone and alprazolam in the clinic. I was going through a rough patch and instead of drinking I just started taking the samples. I liked the way they made me feel and it wasn't long before I started increasing the quantity of these drugs I was ordering from my wholesale distributor to cover what I needed for my addiction in addition to what we needed for the practice."

Many physicians in solo or small group practice have access to massive quantities of prescription medications through distributors. Some addicted physicians have had controlled prescription medications, never intended for patient use, delivered directly to their homes and stored in their garages. As licensed practitioners they are responsible for strict accounting and safe storage of medications in order to protect the public from diversion of these potentially dangerous substances, but addicted healthcare professionals care about little else other than access to these medications for personal use.

Because of the high risk for abuse and addiction associated with these medications, stimulants containing amphetamines and methylphenidate are prescribed for only a few conditions, most commonly ADHD, narcolepsy and refractory depression. These drugs come in pill form and are either taken orally or crushed, dissolved in water and injected. Healthcare professionals have been known to abuse these medications most often for their "performance enhancement" properties which allow students to remain awake and alert during long periods of study and residents or other shift workers to remain vigilant during extended periods of duty.

First the Professionals, Then the Rest of Us

It is not only the healthcare professionals who have ready access to prescription drugs who are abusing them. Prescription drug abuse is a growing problem across all populations, especially in younger people. The Drug Abuse Warning Network (DAWN) monitors medications and illicit drugs reported in emergency departments across the United States. Data obtained from persons who required emergency treatment for prescription drug-related issues suggest that the levels of this type of drug abuse escalated during the late 1990s, with the greatest increase in users ages twelve to twenty-one.[4]

Emergency room visits caused by narcotic pain medications increased 350 percent during the period from 1994 to 2002, with the most frequently reported prescription medications in these drug abuse-related cases being the narcotic pain relievers oxycodone, hydrocodone, morphine and methadone.[5] From 1994 to 2002, ERs reveal hydrocodone and oxycodone increased by 170 percent and 450 percent, respectively.[6] But it is not only narcotic medications that are causing people to end up in the ER requiring emergency treatment. The frequency with which patients are presenting with overdoses from prescription CNS depressant drugs, benzodiazepines such as diazepam, alprazolam, clonazepam and lorazepam, is also increasing. These drugs are being used frequently in combination with other drugs of abuse, an often deadly combination.[7] This evidence of increased use reflects the increased availability of these medications for abuse by medical personnel as well as by the general public.

For the most part, prescription drugs are obtained from a friend or relative who was legitimately prescribed them and then either gave them away or sold them. But users who want these increasingly popular drugs can also get them from dealers or directly from physicians who either unwittingly or willingly write prescriptions. "Doctor shopping," in which an addict will go from one physician to the next presenting the same symptoms and asking for prescription drugs, is less common in younger generations of users who are more likely to obtain these drugs from friends with access, often to wholesale quantities of these medications via Internet pharmacies.

With increasing frequency, these drugs are stolen, often from pharmacies in dramatic armed robberies. Medical personnel have unique access to these drugs and it is this access, coupled with an intimate knowledge of how these drugs work and an increasing familiarity with recreational use, that has contributed to a rise in abuse in the medical professional population. It seems that prescription drug abuse is a fact of life for today's new medical professionals, much as illicit drug abuse was a fact of life for prior generations.

Today, a young person who begins to use drugs is just as likely to use marijuana as a prescription medication. Younger healthcare workers are more likely to have been exposed to increased recreational use of pharmaceuticals either themselves or among friends or classmates. One survey of college students in 2005 reported that 3.1 percent had abused painkillers such as oxycodone, in either immediate release or extended release preparations, and hydrocodone during the previous month, up from less than 1 percent of students in 1993.[8] This increase reflects the increasing availability of prescription drugs used recreationally in this population. As of 2008, the average age for first nonmedical use of prescription drugs was twenty-two years old, the age when today's new medical, dental and nursing students, resident physicians and emergency medical personnel are entering the workforce.[9]

It is no great surprise that the increased abuse of these medications observed in the general population has carried over to the population of young healthcare professionals. In many cases, the natural history of the abused prescription drug can be traced to prescriber abuse long before the general public got ahold of it. Perhaps the overall increase in prescription drug abuse is a reflection of this increase in provider drug abuse. I strongly believe that if the epidemic starts with the healthcare professional first, then this is where it should be stopped.

PART III

PROTECTING YOURSELF FROM ADDICTED HEALTHCARE PROFESSIONALS

CHAPTER 7

Identifying Addicted Healthcare Professionals

How do you know if your doctor is using drugs? What can you look for if you suspect your nurse might be stealing drugs from you or your loved one? Could your dentist be high? What about the emergency medical personnel, laboratory technicians, pharmacists and ancillary healthcare professionals you may only come in contact with on rare occasions? Early identification of addicted professionals can prevent harm to both the addicted healthcare providers and their patients, but this is not an easy task.[1]

We live such compartmentalized lives that the entire picture is seldom seen by any one person. Friends and family members of addicted healthcare professionals may notice changes at home that they may attribute to work-related stress and colleagues at work may attribute these changes to problems at home. This is especially true for healthcare professionals who work long shifts and may not see their friends or families over an extended period of time. Patients who have limited contact with their healthcare providers may not notice subtle changes in behavior.

Paramedic, Husband, Heroin Addict

Addicted healthcare professionals present with a wide range of severity of the signs and symptoms suggestive of drug use. John, a paramedic, reported casual but regular use of intravenous narcotics. "I work twenty-four hour shifts on the rigs. When I come home, I sleep; then I go back to work. Sometimes after a long shift it's hard to get to sleep. I'll use some morphine so I can crash before the next shift." Even though he cannot prescribe these substances himself, as a paramedic John has access to morphine and other potent intravenous pain medications. At times he administers these drugs to patients en route to the hospital under the orders of an emergency medicine physician. "When we get a patient who's having a heart attack or has been involved in a motor vehicle accident and needs these medications, we contact the base station and the ER doc at the hospital where we're headed gives me the authorization to administer the drugs."

The narcotics are in a locked box in the ambulance and accounting is taken at the beginning and end of each shift, but it's easy to skim some off the top. "If I want to I can say that I gave the morphine to a patient and then keep it for myself." John admitted that occasionally he takes street drugs from his patients and keeps them for himself. "Sometimes it's easier just to take something off a junkie who's overdosed. There's much less chance of getting caught. It's not like I'm the police or anything. I don't care what they've been doing and it's not like they're going to say, 'Hey, that medic stole my drugs' or anything like that, though sometimes they do."

Despite the existence of programs designed to treat affected individuals, denial, shame, guilt and fear may play a role in preventing addicted healthcare professionals from seeking help until very late in the disease. John doesn't think he has a problem with drugs, but he is in denial. Denial can make identification and subsequent treatment of addicted healthcare professionals very difficult, as addicted individuals often do not even recognize that a problem exists. These are generally well-educated, highly functioning people with well-developed defense mechanisms and grandiose ideas of invulnerability and self-sufficiency. They very rarely seek treatment on their own as they are unable to accept that their drug use cannot be controlled and will ultimately lead to addiction. Because of this, it is essential that the people closest to healthcare professionals know what to look for and understand what to do when they discover a problem.

Denial is not limited to the addict. Coworkers, friends, relatives and associates presented with behavior that clearly suggests an addiction problem exists will often make excuses for an addicted healthcare professional. While it can be difficult to accept that a problem is the result of addiction, the identification of specific behavior patterns suggestive of abuse, culminating in a properly executed intervention, can save the life of an addicted healthcare professional as well as prevent significant harm to patients.[2]

John is involved in a long-term relationship with Beth, who is also a paramedic. "We started dating when we were partners at work. I was married and John was dating someone, but with the long hours together, you very quickly develop a bond. It can be very intense and during the slow times there's a 'bed' in the back of the rig so it's easy to have sex."

Even though they no longer work on the same shift, Beth and John probably see each other more often at work than at home. "We come and go at different times, so it's easier to meet up while we're both out. Sometimes I'll come home while I'm on duty and he's always passed out or something." When asked whether she thinks John has a problem with drugs, Beth hedges. "He probably uses more than he should, but it doesn't really affect his performance at work. I remember getting a call from John while I was at work and having to go home and give him naloxone (a narcotic antagonist used to reverse the effects of a narcotic overdose). He had taken some heroin off a junkie who overdosed the day before and then he shot up while I was at work. Apparently, it was some really good stuff. He wanted to enjoy the rush again and didn't want to come down first, so he called me home to bring the naloxone."

Self-identification of addiction is rare but it may occur in the setting of therapy begun for another reason, such as couples therapy or treatment for depression or anxiety. Perhaps if John and Beth were able to address John's drug use directly with the help of a therapist, Beth might be able to overcome her own denial. Despite her protestations, it is likely that John's regular drug use is affecting his performance on the job and it is only a matter of time before someone gets hurt because of it. If the problem of addiction is not identified and treated early in the course of the disease, social or family dysfunction will worsen and work performance will eventually suffer, putting patients at risk for misdiagnosis or injury.

Recognizing the Signs of Addiction

Unlike a civilian addict whose pursuit of his drug of choice often prevents him from participating in productive activities, addicted healthcare providers may appear rather functional until the very end of their addictions. As other parts of their lives are left to fall apart, addicted healthcare providers struggle to maintain jobs close to their sources of drugs. An addicted anesthesia care professional may volunteer for additional evening and weekend assignments or for long cases in which large narcotic requirements would be expected. An addicted nurse may accept overtime shifts in patient care areas where administration of controlled drugs is routine.

There are multiple reasons that healthcare professionals exhibit these behaviors that could be entirely unrelated to substance abuse. Primary among them is a need to increase personal income or a desire to advance one's career or establish a reputation in a particular area. It is not the behaviors so much as the changes in behavior that should arouse suspicion. Here are the five key changes typically observed in individuals affected by prescription drug abuse:

Five Key Signs a Healthcare Professional May be Drug Impaired

1. Changes in personal behavior:
   - Withdrawal from family, friends and leisure activities
   - Deterioration of interpersonal relations

2. Mood swings:
   - Periods of depression (while in withdrawal) alternating with periods of euphoria (while intoxicated)
   - Characterized by increased episodes of anger, irritability and hostility

3. Changes to personal appearance:
   - Unexplained weight loss
   - Pale skin
   - Unkempt or unprofessional appearance for someone who previously took pride in his or her appearance

- Wearing long sleeves when inappropriate (in order to hide evidence of intravenous injections)

4. Increasing unreliability:
   - Missing appointments or deadlines
   - Increasing number of performance errors, mistakes or oversights
   - Inability to accept blame or admit mistakes
   - Confusion or difficulty concentrating on ordinary tasks which seem to take more time than they should

5. Inappropriate prescriptions:
   - Writing for controlled drugs for personal use
   - Asking patients to fill prescriptions for the professional

Changes Related to Professional Behavior

- Spending more time at the hospital, even when off duty (to remain close to the supply of drugs)
- Volunteering for extra on call or overtime shifts
- A fluctuating level of productivity
- Performance suffers from mistakes or oversights
- Refusing relief for lunch or coffee breaks (so that drugs can be diverted for personal use)
- Requesting frequent bathroom breaks (so these drugs can be used)
- Signing out increasing amounts of narcotics or wasting increasing quantities
- Insisting on personally administering controlled drugs
- Inappropriate prescriptions for controlled drugs

How long does it take for these changes in addicted individuals to become evident? It depends on the drug to which an individual has become addicted. While addiction to alcohol typically takes years to produce changes that significantly interfere with an individual's ability to compensate, addiction to short-acting narcotics like fentanyl and sufentanil becomes apparent over the course of a few months of use. What starts out as casual or occasional use very quickly becomes a regular habit.

Before individuals are even aware of what is going on, they have become physically dependent on the medications and need them in higher quantities and more frequently. If they don't get the medications they need, they begin to feel cravings for the drugs and recreational or social activities that once occupied a good portion of the individuals' free time fall by the wayside as the only activity that matters is obtaining and using more of the drugs. Healthcare professionals who are abusing prescription medications will let relations with friends and family languish, as they no longer have the ability to focus on anyone or anything other than the drugs they need. All of this can occur in a relatively short period of time, which is why looking for changes in behavior is just as important as looking at the behaviors themselves.

Not an Isolated Case

Denial is not limited to the addicts. Often, in retrospect, family members, coworkers and friends admit that they knew something was wrong, but they didn't want to say anything. There is a natural reluctance to talk about this subject. Maybe the people involved with the addicts didn't want to risk angering the addicts or feared retribution; maybe they didn't want to damage their colleagues' careers or perhaps jeopardize their licenses. Maybe admitting the truth was too difficult, so instead they made excuses for behavior which, in hindsight, represented addiction. Our society currently supports a great legal machine, the implications of which are far-reaching and affect medical care in often unintended ways.

The evidence of this litigiousness can be seen in the multiple dramatic commercials for law firms willing to help injured healthcare consumers obtain financial compensation for medical malpractice and which are aired throughout the day, presumably when the injured individuals who cannot work would be watching television. Doctors now order tests, laboratory work and intervention that may not be necessary but to make sure they are covered in the event of a lawsuit. The idea that any infraction may ultimately result in litigation has driven the creation of policy which, while claiming to embrace openness and full disclosure, suffocates patients' rights for information about the quality of their treatment. As a result, the friends, family members and coworkers who are unwilling to become involved and open themselves up to potential legal action become enablers, allowing addicted healthcare professionals to continue to put themselves and their patients in harm's way.

Marc is an anesthesiologist at an academic program in New England. "Last year, when I found a vial of fentanyl that nobody reported missing, I knew someone was diverting. I work in the cardiac operating rooms where we spill more fentanyl on the floor in a given day than most use for a day's worth of cases in the general operating rooms, but nobody is going to misplace a twenty milliliter bullet." I asked Marc what he did when he discovered the vial. "I turned it in to the pharmacy, of course, but nobody reported missing it." Marc didn't report his suspicions that one of his colleagues or one of the residents was diverting fentanyl. "I didn't want to be wrong. I figured if someone was using that much fentanyl that they would be discovered soon anyway and I didn't want to get involved." As it turned out, one of the residents had been diverting fentanyl and was discovered eight weeks later. When asked how he would have felt if this resident had turned up dead, Marc quickly replied, "It's not my business."

Marc's decision not to become involved is an example of the culture of acceptance and denial that allows self-medication and other forms of drug use to continue past the point where patients' lives are put at risk. Physicians are told that, just as the lawyer who represents himself has a fool for a client, the doctor who treats himself or his family is receiving substandard care. Historically, professional courtesy has been extended from one physician to another in recognition of this and there are still some who do not charge or offer discounts to other physicians. However, as reimbursements for professional services continue to be cut, it is hard for those who can treat themselves or their families to resist the temptation to do so. When medical professionals see suspect behavior, they often look the other way. This has to stop.

The special circumstances that confound identification of addicted healthcare professionals place the responsibility on those who have regular contact with these individuals. Coworkers, friends and family are most likely to be the first ones to spot the behavior changes discussed. By the time an addicted healthcare professional has deteriorated to the point where his or her addiction becomes obvious to the casual observer, it has likely been obvious to those who have had regular contact for some time. The behaviors described are typical of any individual addicted to any drug, but it is more than being able to recognize behavior patterns or changes.

In order to help, you will have to be able to work through the denial or doubt that your friend, family member or colleague might be using drugs and address the issue. Given the increasing number of persons who become addicted to prescription medications each year, it is likely only a matter of time until you find yourself in a situation where this information becomes critical. Given the high motivation for licensed healthcare professionals to maintain their ability to practice, gentile coercion into treatment is often all that is necessary to begin the healing process. While there are unlimited reasons or excuses you can come up with to explain away suspect behavior, you only need to come up with one reason to help.

Chapter 8

Reporting Impaired Healthcare Professionals

A s we have seen, addiction to drugs and alcohol can interfere with healthcare professionals' ability to practice competently and puts the general public at risk for injury. At the very least, impaired physicians, nurses and other healthcare workers provide substandard care when they are either under the influence or in withdrawal. In its worst manifestation, patient death or severe injury is possible. The need to identify and remove impaired healthcare professionals from positions where they could potentially cause harm may seem obvious, but even after identification has occurred, reporting these individuals still presents a challenge. We exist in a culture which, to some degree, gives a subtle wink and a nod to recreational drug use and the healthcare professionals among us can benefit from this sly complicity.

At the same time, healthcare professionals understand that when they chose to become providers of care they would be held to a higher standard than the rest of the population. Because of the considerable stigma still attached to addiction and the high stakes associated with such an accusation, the coworkers of an addicted individual are often unwilling to put this matter forward for investigation until very late in the disease. Colleagues often can identify with an addicted healthcare professional, even if they themselves do not misuse drugs.

Being unwilling to voice such a concern lest they are wrong or accused of slander, they keep their observations to themselves. This form of denial is the manifestation of a very well-developed defense mechanism in healthcare workers who witness trauma and misery on a regular basis and must push this reality toward the back of their minds so that they can focus on treating the sick and dying.

Because addicted healthcare professionals, through their drug using behaviors, have put the lives and safety of others who depend on them at significant risk for death and injury, it can be hard to find sympathy for these individuals. It is important to remember, however, that addiction is a disease and that these people are ill and in as much need of treatment as the patients for whom they care. As we learn the stories of what these people have done and what they have gone through, it is important to keep in mind that addicts are also suffering human beings who need care and compassion. In order to function in a world filled with pain and misery, healthcare professionals must distance themselves from the reality of their professions; for some people this means turning to drugs. Addicted healthcare professionals are at very real risk for injury or death due to the nature of the medications to which they have become addicted.

Reporting an impaired healthcare professional can not only prevent injury to future patients but also prevent very serious injury or death to the addict as well. In many cases, bringing this issue to light can also change the culture of an institution such as a hospital or physician's practice which has allowed this behavior to flourish. The persistent false belief that addiction is the result of moral weakness and not a disease, which is so deeply ingrained in our culture, does not allow one to voice publicly what, in retrospect, was obvious to most. Perhaps a shift in the perception of what addiction really is might make more addicted healthcare professionals ask for help or enter treatment on their own.

Change is difficult and a lot of inertia exists, which makes adjustment of our attitudes difficult, but this would be a great step toward increasing patient safety. Given the current attitudes that society has regarding the disease of addiction, it is surprising that any impaired healthcare professionals end up in treatment before patient harm occurs. So what, if anything, can you do if you suspect your physician or nurse is using drugs?

An Addict with Excellent Recommendations

Dr. Robert Berry worked as an anesthesiologist at a number of different locations over the course of several years before he ended up at his current medical center. While it is not common for anesthesiologists in practice to move from one job to another on a regular basis, it is not unheard of and the due diligence performed by the medical center staff that hired Dr. Berry turned up nothing to suggest that he was anything other than competent and fit for duty. He had, in fact, received two positive letters of recommendation from physician colleagues at his former employer's group and it is unlikely that the hiring staff was aware that it had hired an addict.[1]

Dr. Berry had worked as an employee of an anesthesia associates group. An investigation into the undocumented removal of meperidine from hospital supplies revealed that Dr. Berry may have been responsible for diversion of this drug. His professional use of meperidine was subsequently monitored for five months and, in March, after he did not respond to a page and was found unfit to work, he was fired.

He was not reported to the hospital's impaired professionals committee, nor was he reported to the state medical board. He was not referred for treatment. Additionally, when they were asked by the medical center to comment on Dr. Berry's past performance relating to an application for credentialing and future employment, representatives of the anesthesia associates group did not disclose any negative information. Furthermore, two physicians still employed by the group wrote positive letters of recommendation which also failed to mention Dr. Berry's addiction problems.

So the medical center hired Dr. Berry and he continued to practice. Apparently he also continued to divert and self-administer meperidine and to care for patients while under the influence of this highly potent and addictive narcotic. Shortly after being hired for this new position, Dr. Berry was involved in an incident which left a young, otherwise healthy woman in a permanent vegetative state. After what was essentially a routine outpatient procedure, Dr. Berry brought his patient to the recovery room. He had given her what he felt was an appropriate dose of narcotic pain medication but removed her breathing tube prematurely and failed to notice that she was not breathing on her own. By the time the nurse in the recovery room realized what was happening, it was too late. Dr. Berry's patient suffered a cardiac arrest, because she did not have enough oxygen. It is likely that any one of several basic maneuvers could have been performed to prevent this from happening. Had Dr. Berry been more vigilant and had he not been impaired through his use of prescription narcotics, things would likely have turned out differently for this patient.

Dr. Robert Berry was found to be responsible for this post-surgical catastrophe and he subsequently admitted that he had been addicted to and under the influence of meperidine at the time. Since this incident occurred while Dr. Berry was an employee of the medical center, the center was found to be liable for damages as well. In an attempt to recover these damages, the medical center sued the anesthesia associates group for intentional misrepresentation of Dr. Berry's fitness to practice medicine. After all, the center argued, it had hired this anesthesiologist partially on the strength of the recommendations from his former employer.

Should the anesthesia associates group have reported Dr. Berry to the state medical board for suspicion of meperidine diversion? Was the group obligated to report such concerns or suspicions to any future employers? The employer felt strongly enough about the evidence suggesting Dr. Berry was diverting meperidine that it terminated his employment for cause. The Court determined that the letters of recommendation from the two physicians, though they did not contain any outright misrepresentations, were false. The Court also determined that the letter from the anesthesia associates group was not misleading, though it did fail to adequately answer the questions that the medical center asked.

Despite the admission by the Court that a possible ethical obligation to disclose Dr. Berry's drug addiction may exist, they did not find that the anesthesia associates group had any legal obligation to do so. Even more troubling was the suggestion that had the group provided negative information that resulted in Dr. Berry not obtaining credentials, it might be liable for defamation. The suggestion that revealing information such as addiction would leave a reference or organization open to legal action sets a very dangerous precedent. The law should serve to shield persons who come forward with such information rather than dissuade them from sharing it. Providing legal protection would serve to protect the public and suggesting the opposite does little to further patient safety issues.

Dr. Berry's case is just one of many examples where impaired physicians and other healthcare professionals have been let go from their employment, because their group did not want to deal with addressing their addiction problems. It appears that employers feel it is much easier to send someone along to find another job and if providing a positive letter of recommendation makes it that much more likely that the addict will go away, then many are tempted to do just that.

The United States Supreme Court refused to hear the appeal of the *Kadlec Medical Center v. Lakeview Anesthesia Associates* decision, effectively supporting the ruling that healthcare providers do not have a legal obligation to disclose information regarding another healthcare professional's drug use.[2]

Isolated or Chronic Event

Given this reluctance for colleagues to come forward and the lack of any legal requirement to do so or legal support if they do, it is more likely that an impaired healthcare professional will come to the attention of authorities through their interaction with the system late in the course of their disease. Depending on the state in which a healthcare professional practices, the law may actually require that when a physician or other healthcare professional is arrested for a criminal offense, he or she is reported to the state licensing body. This is not the standard everywhere, however, so it is still possible that physicians charged with assault, rape or possibly even murder might be able to continue to practice medicine until convicted. At the other end of the spectrum are the states in the United States and places around the world that have much stricter reporting policies. In some states, drunk driving or driving while under the influence of drugs is considered to be unprofessional conduct, an offense reportable to the state licensing board.

These reports are investigated to determine if it is an isolated incident or reflects an underlying issue that has the potential to cause patient harm. Since the primary function of the state licensing boards is to protect the public, they are more likely to move forward with disciplinary action and will err on the side of caution when choosing between the license of a potentially impaired healthcare practitioner and public safety, but not always. Not every state requires mandatory reporting of impaired healthcare professionals if patient harm has not occurred and many such individuals opt to enter treatment voluntarily, thereby completely avoiding contact with the licensing board.

Rarely is an impaired healthcare professional reported by someone who is not involved in the medical profession. Typically this comes as the result of some incident related to substandard care or patient injury or it may be something as simple as a family member reporting the smell of alcohol on the breath of the surgeon caring for a loved one.

Dr. James, a pediatric surgeon, continues to work while in treatment for addiction to alcohol. "I'm the only surgeon they have, so my job involves being on call pretty much all the time. The hospital needs me around, because I'm the only pediatric surgeon who can do these procedures." Dr. James came to the attention of the authorities not because of any adverse event related to substandard patient care, but because he was reported by the parents of one of his patients.

"It was an evening a few years back when my wife and I had gone over to a friend's house for dinner. Even though I was technically on call, it was a Friday night and I hadn't done an emergency case in the evening for months. Wouldn't you know I had a couple of drinks and then my pager goes off?" Dr. James was called to the hospital to care for a ten-year-old who had suffered a traumatic bladder injury. The procedure went well and, after the surgery, he went to the waiting area to discuss the prognosis with the child's parents. "The conversation went well, but I could tell the father was suspicious of something. At the end, he pulled me aside and let me know that he was a state trooper and that he could smell the alcohol on my breath." As a result of this report Dr. James is now involved in a treatment and monitoring program.

Making a Report

The public has two avenues available for reporting potentially impaired licensed healthcare professionals. If malpractice has occurred, a person may file a lawsuit. To prevail, the person would then have to prove that the healthcare professional in question had a duty to the patient, that the professional breached that duty, that an injury occurred and that this injury was caused by the healthcare professional's breach of duty.

But what about the obligation or desire to report the impaired healthcare professional when harm has not occurred? Some people believe strongly that an obligation to do so exists despite the current case law and have proposed that victims of medical malpractice should be able to recover damages from a former employer who failed to disclose information that could have prevented the injury from occurring. Other options for reporting exist, however, and can be used to file a complaint directly with the licensing board. Dr. Kramer, the radiologist turned medi-spa operator whom we focused on earlier, was reported through the same mechanism available to the public and it is quite possible that, even though this report was not without an ulterior motive on the part of the facialist, patient health and safety were advanced.

If you believe a healthcare professional is impaired and represents an imminent danger to him or herself or to others, you can file a direct report anonymously through the state medical or nursing board as appropriate or via direct contact with the state medical or nursing society.

CHAPTER 9

Legal Issues and Addicted Healthcare Professionals

The drugs that healthcare professionals most often become addicted to have legitimate medical uses, which presents a special problem when it comes to regulation of these medications. Historically, limiting the healthcare community's ability to use medications with significant abuse potential by criminalizing their misuse or holding physicians and other healthcare providers accountable for the actions of their patients has had a chilling effect. Healthcare professionals, fearing retribution from law enforcement, have decreased use of some medications, leading to the inadequate treatment of pain and needless human suffering.

As a result of this unintended consequence, in recent years legislation has swung in the opposite direction and some physicians have been successfully sued for under-treatment of pain. I personally believe that a balance needs to be maintained between the reasonable prohibition against inappropriate use of these substances and laws which effectively prevent their use entirely. It is not acceptable to punish legitimate use of these medications or limit access to them through draconian legislation drafted in response to public demand that "something has to be done."

Addiction in the healthcare setting presents a special problem, however, as these people are responsible for the health and well-being of all members of society. Patients trust that every healthcare professional will do his or her best to ensure that no harm will come to them, even during the most minor procedures, but when healthcare professionals are addicts, either under the influence of drugs or in withdrawal from them, this cannot happen.

Current legal policy reflects the necessity to balance the needs of society with the rights of the addicted practitioner. As the addiction epidemic continues to unfold and touches the lives of more and more people, the public demand for political leaders to take action will undoubtedly approach crisis level. It is essential that lawmakers not enact inappropriate, reactionary legislation that does not take into consideration the unintended consequences of unnecessarily punitive laws.

The response of the legal community regarding the issue of impaired healthcare professionals has become a vigorous and growing one, with legal battles raging in the courtroom and on Capitol Hill. The policy issues being debated today will become the laws which will shape the healthcare community's response to this growing problem in years to come. As we consider how we are going to address this epidemic, it is essential to remember that addiction is a disease and needs to be treated as such. While the primary policy goal should be to protect the public, we cannot forget that these healthcare professionals are also members of our society and deserve just as much protection and treatment. Addicted healthcare professionals should be removed from positions where they could potentially harm themselves or someone else, undergo effective treatment and rehabilitation and, when appropriate, return to clinical practice.

Legislation Affecting Impaired Healthcare Professionals

Public recognition of the issue of addiction in the healthcare professionals population began with the publication of "The Sick Physician" report by the American Medical Association (AMA) in the 1970s.[1] This report brought to the forefront the issue of the impaired physician and made policy recommendations designed to address this issue, including the creation of treatment programs for physicians impaired through their addictions to drugs and alcohol. Though the AMA specifically addressed the issue of the impaired physician, the natural extension of such a policy was to address the impaired healthcare professional in general, regardless of occupation.

Recognition that nurses, dentists, pharmacists and any one of the professionals involved with the delivery of healthcare could develop the disease of addiction and deserve treatment within the context of this policy has driven the expansion of physician-only treatment programs to include greater numbers and types of healthcare professionals. This move away from a policy of ignoring these issues or dealing with the addicted healthcare provider through punitive measures and toward policy focused on treatment and rehabilitation has culminated in the creation of the impaired professionals programs currently active in most locations. Patient safety has seen a direct benefit from this shift in attitudes, as impaired healthcare professionals are more likely to seek treatment proactively today than in the past when such programs were not available.

In 1989, the Oregon State Senate passed Senate Bill 1032, establishing the Diversion Program Supervisory Council, which specified the structure and funding for what was the first statewide impaired physician program.[2] Since the creation of this program, the remaining forty-nine states have followed Oregon's lead and established similar programs for physicians, though some of the less effective programs have either closed or been turned over to private management.[3] Programs specifically designed to address the issue of addicted nurses and other healthcare professionals have followed, but not in every state. One need look no further than the impaired nurses programs for an example of why this policy change is so important in protecting both the addicted healthcare professionals and the patients for whom they care. In states that do not offer alternatives to discipline programs but instead respond to any accusation of impairment with punitive measures, the potentially impaired nurse remains in practice much longer than in states where the carrot of rehabilitation and return to clinical practice is available. Since the goal of any such program should be to protect both the patient and the provider, the policy which gets the addict out of the clinical setting and into treatment sooner is the better one.

Legislation and policy has also been designed to address the issue of impaired healthcare professionals who come in contact with the law for nonmedical reasons. An addicted healthcare professional is less likely than a civilian addict to encounter law enforcement personnel through the procurement of drugs since this is rarely a street crime. Most addicted healthcare professionals are not buying their drugs from dealers in a back alley; in many cases they can purchase their drugs directly from manufacturers. Possible involvement with the Drug Enforcement Agency occurs when diversion is recognized and reported to law enforcement, although, by the time this happens, a healthcare professional is frequently in the intervention process or already in treatment.

It is more likely that an addicted healthcare professional will encounter law enforcement personnel in the context of being under the influence while away from work, usually while operating a motor vehicle or involved in fights, domestic altercations or public intoxication. For most people, an arrest for one of these drug-related offenses does not trigger a call to one's employer, but for a healthcare professional it might.

Some states make it a matter of policy or law to have the police inform the professional board when such a professional is convicted of any criminal offense. Other states extend this policy to include an arrest for any infraction with the understanding that the board will sort out the issues and determine if this is an isolated incident or represents a symptom of a much larger problem. Still other states require notification only in the case of an arrest or conviction involving crimes of moral turpitude, such as those involving the distribution or sale of controlled substances or operating a motor vehicle while under the influence. The penalties handed down for such infractions by law enforcement are invariably harsher than the penalties imposed by the board. In most cases, a healthcare professional who runs afoul of the law is much more likely to receive a summons and legal sanctions than he is to receive action or even a reprimand from the licensing board.

Legal Protections Afforded Addicted Healthcare Professionals

The Americans with Disabilities Act (ADA) offers some protections to addicted healthcare providers, placing the responsibility on the employer to prove that an employee is unable to perform the responsibilities of his occupation. According to the act, "No covered entity shall discriminate against a qualified individual on the basis of disability in regard to job application procedures, the hiring, advancement, or discharge of employees, employee compensation, job training, and other terms, conditions, and privileges of employment."[4] These protections are limited in scope and have been applied differently to individuals who are dependent upon alcohol versus illegal (or legal) drugs.[5]

To establish protection under this act, a healthcare professional must first prove that he or she is disabled within the definition of the act. Some courts have found that alcoholism or substance abuse itself is not necessarily a disability under the ADA definition and no protection has been afforded to a user of substances other than alcohol unless he is currently in a treatment or monitoring program.

Regardless of how disability is defined, if an impaired healthcare professional is treated as though he or she is disabled, if he or she is offered treatment instead of termination when found to be addicted, then the professional is considered disabled and the terms of the act apply.[6] This protection extends both to employment within the context of treatment and to subsequent applications for employment or license renewal. Should an impaired healthcare professional be fired for cause, having been found to have violated a zero-tolerance no-drug workplace policy, the professional would not be afforded this protection.

A healthcare professional who is found to be addicted to drugs and is offered the opportunity to enter a treatment program, however, cannot subsequently be relieved of his or her duties solely on the basis of his or her status as a recovering addict once he or she successfully completes such a program, provided the professional is not under the influence. To fire such an individual because he or she is in recovery from addiction would be a violation of the protections afforded by the ADA and would leave the employer liable should the individual choose to sue for discrimination.

The protection against discrimination based on disability further extends to pre-employment questioning regarding previous experience with impairment. The ADA specifically prohibits employers from asking questions about the nature and extent of a disability during the pre-employment interview, based on the grounds that such questions are intrusive and require disclosure of protected personal health information. A physician or nurse in recovery who is applying for a new clinical position is often required to sign an affidavit attesting to the fact that he or she does not have any condition or disability that would interfere with his or her ability to discharge the duties of the position for which he or she is applying and that he or she does not use drugs or alcohol illegally. Such attestations are carefully worded to avoid conflicts with the ADA and to allow a healthcare professional in recovery to answer truthfully in the affirmative. Such pre-employment questionnaires also include questions such as current or past (within the last five years for example) involvement with an impaired professionals monitoring program, though an affirmative answer cannot be grounds to deny employment to an otherwise qualified applicant.

The protections afforded to the healthcare professional in recovery by the ADA do not specifically apply to either the licensing or credentialing process and individual states may or may not ask questions about prior experience with addiction. Some state medical boards require an attestation for any physician who is currently involved in a monitoring program that he or she is not impaired and remains free from the influence of drugs, legal or otherwise. Other state medical boards require notification but no attestation, while other states seem to have a "don't ask, don't tell" policy when it comes to this issue. Diversion of controlled substances is, however, a felony, and if charges are brought, the ADA does not offer any protection.

Impaired Practitioner Policies

Recognizing that an impaired healthcare professional lacks the ability to care for patients safely and that this represents an institutional liability, hospitals must have a policy in place designed to protect patients and addicted professionals. The most appropriate policy is a zero-tolerance policy which does not allow any employee to abuse drugs and/or alcohol at any time. It makes sense that an employer wouldn't want an employee to work while intoxicated, but because of the nature of the drugs we have been discussing, it makes sense to prohibit their use during time away from work for any employee. Typically these policies are designed to cover a wide range of impairment, including physical or mental illness which impairs cognitive or motor skills, but the majority of the cases involve the use of alcohol or drugs. For this purpose most institutions define "drug" to include alcohol, illegal drugs such as cocaine, heroin or marijuana and legal drugs with legitimate medical uses.

The content of such policies varies across institutions and different states have differing legal precedents, but all have the same aims: to empower any member of the institutional staff to report suspicion of substance abuse or impairment by providing legal protection for reports made in good faith and clearly outlining what steps should be taken by the institution when such a report is made. Such policies must clearly state that reporting impaired healthcare professionals is a patient safety issue and is the responsibility of every member of the healthcare team. In the event that such impairment is reported, certain issues must be addressed:

- **To whom should the report be made?**
  Sometimes the direct supervisor is responsible for receiving such information but frequently there is a medical review officer or member of the impaired professionals committee in charge of handling these issues. It is particularly important to follow procedures properly when the impaired professional is a senior physician or high-level institutional executive. Since these reports are often made after hours, an on call individual should be available to receive evening or weekend reports and this person should be responsible for determining the course of the investigation and what steps are called for.

- **What is the policy regarding the collection of samples for drug testing?**
  This is a very sensitive issue and should be covered in detail by the institutional drug testing policy. When an

investigation into an allegation of impairment due to drugs or alcohol requires a sample for analysis (usually urine, blood or hair as outlined by the policy), the collection of said sample should be conducted with as much confidentiality as possible while still observing all witnessed collection protocols and ensuring that the chain of custody record is maintained. It is of the upmost importance that the initial specimen collection is performed under the strictest adherence to forensic policy. The sample collection should be witnessed by two individuals and sealed in a container with a non-resealable closure and evidentiary tape to ensure against tampering. This specimen should then be transported with a paper chain of custody log and split prior to analysis so that part of the initial unassayed sample remains for confirmatory testing. It is important to identify, prior to testing, what prescription or over-the-counter drugs the healthcare professional has been taking for legitimate reasons so that the test results can be interpreted in the proper context. Many institutions consider the refusal to provide a sample as an admission of drug use.

- **What do you do with the healthcare professional while you are waiting for the results of the drug test?**
It should be the intent of the institution to maintain the safety of both the impaired healthcare practitioner as well as the patients. In this light, it is often prudent to suspend the individual's clinical privileges or duties for a reasonable period of time, so that an investigation can be performed pending the outcome of any sample analysis. This investigation should be performed as quickly as is reasonable so as not to disrupt any patient care activities or delay admission to a treatment program for the impaired professional.

- **What if the test is positive?**
Depending upon institutional policy, healthcare professionals who test positive may have their employment terminated or they may be given a temporary leave of absence

so that they may attend a rehabilitation program, after which privileges or employment may be reinstated. This policy should be made clear to all employees at the time that they begin working at the institution so that everyone understands what will happen if someone is found to have been using drugs while working.

• **What if the healthcare professional wants to appeal the test results?**
  Occasionally a positive test result is contested. If the practitioner wishes to have an independent laboratory assay the sample and correct procedures were followed for collecting the original sample, then part of the sample remains available for further testing.

• **What happens to a healthcare professional who is determined to have been impaired?**
  If the medical review officer determines that the healthcare professional in question is impaired or if there is any question, the professional should be referred to either the state medical or nursing society or the appropriate impaired professionals program for further evaluation or treatment.

When lives are potentially at stake, it can be hard to accept that due process remains paramount, but when you look at the "big picture" view it becomes clear. Addicted healthcare professionals have often backed themselves into a corner and may see no safe way out of their current situations. Because they are acutely aware that discovery will potentially cost them their careers, their livelihoods and in some cases their freedom, these people will do anything to avoid being caught.

The legal protections and policies discussed in this chapter were drafted with the intent of protecting the public. Also inherent in this process is protecting the addicts. Without hope there is only despair and when addicted healthcare professionals find their careers in jeopardy, they may fight treatment rather than surrender to the process of recovery.

As we will see in the next section, by providing legal protections and alternatives to discipline programs which allow impaired practitioners to enter treatment voluntarily in exchange for leniency or a stay of revocation by the medical or nursing board, addicted healthcare professionals are removed from patient contact sooner than they otherwise would be. Patient safety is increased by removing addicted healthcare professionals from clinical settings and getting them into treatment before harm can be done.

PART IV

HELP AND RECOVERY FOR ADDICTED HEALTHCARE PROFESSIONALS

Chapter 10

Treatment Options

Healthcare providers represent a vital human resource essential for our society. There are considerable costs associated with educating healthcare professionals (tuition and living expenses for college, medical or graduate school and advanced training during which these professionals are not in the workforce). Medical education begins in school, but healthcare professionals continue to learn from their experiences, both informally through daily work and formally through mandated updates on medical advances. The seasoned physician or nurse has knowledge and skills that only come with clinical practice and this cannot be taught in school. Addicted healthcare professionals cannot be replaced easily with new graduates as the economic and social costs are too great.

Addiction is a chronic, relapsing disease for which there is no cure, only treatment. In this section, we'll focus on why the addicted healthcare professional is particularly difficult to treat and the reasons why the consequences of relapse are so serious. We will examine the healthcare professionals' treatment program in depth as this program is the gold standard for addiction treatment and should be viewed as a model for all other programs. We will also take a closer look at the programs designed to monitor rehabilitated professionals once they have completed the inpatient portions of their treatments and discuss their prospects for return to clinical practice.

Despite the considerable obstacles to recovery in this population, the evidence suggests that the programs designed to treat healthcare professionals are effective and the initial expenses are well worth it. When coupled with mandatory multi-year monitoring contracts, these professional health programs graduate large numbers of individuals who are capable of remaining drug and alcohol free. Treatment programs have been designed to protect the public while at the same time maximizing the potential for successful return to clinical practice.

Addiction rehabilitation treatment is expensive and financially out of reach for the majority of patients who are not healthcare professionals, but it costs much less than educating a replacement healthcare professional. Even some in the healthcare field may find the price of this mandated treatment to be prohibitive, but the considerable cost in terms of time and financial investment required to participate in such a program is still less than the alternative.

Many in the addiction treatment community consider medical professionals who are addicted difficult to deal with. Addicted healthcare professionals are, in general, highly motivated, highly intelligent individuals who have devoted considerable time, effort and expense to their education and training. They have a lot to lose if their professional licenses are revoked and they can no longer work in their chosen fields. This threat makes them highly motivated to deny that they have done anything that could possibly result in such revocation and loss of livelihood.

Since admission of bad behavior associated with addiction (such as diverting prescription medications for personal use, falsifying medical records or caring for patients while under the influence) is essential for treatment and could result in sanctions imposed by the boards of medicine or nursing, hiding such behaviors can present considerable blocks to recovery. Paradoxically, it is this motivation to keep one's license to practice that is often used to coerce an addicted healthcare professional into a treatment program. Harsh penalties are sometimes imposed but, fortunately, the prognosis for prolonged recovery for most addicted healthcare professionals is excellent, provided they have entered solid treatment programs with proper monitoring.

The overwhelming majority of physician health programs (PHPs)—programs specifically designed to monitor the treatment of addicted physicians—report success rates far in excess of the 50 percent one-year sobriety rates that the programs available to nonmedical personnel typically produce.[1] The most recent data shows that 78 percent of healthcare professionals were able to remain sober and relapse-free five years after completing initial inpatient treatment.[2] Of these, only 22 percent reportedly tested positive for drugs of abuse at any time during their five-year monitoring contract and fully 71 percent remained licensed and employed five years after initial treatment.[3] This is especially impressive given the high relapse rate seen in members of the civilian population who frequently attend much shorter inpatient programs with little or no aftercare. Despite the expense and sacrifice that participating in such a program requires, given their impressive success rates it would be a great benefit to our society if these programs could be made available to all addicted persons, regardless of profession.

Seeking Intervention

The addict is almost always the last to recognize that a problem exists. The people most likely to observe the signs and symptoms of addiction—friends, family members and colleagues—need to have a clear understanding of the disease and what to do if they suspect someone may have a problem. Unfortunately, most addicted healthcare professionals are identified late in their addictions, either when their inability to function at work has become evident or when a crisis such as an overdose occurs.

Each hospital typically assigns individuals familiar with intervention protocol to be responsible for the health and welfare of its workers. These persons should have sufficient information and expertise to assist in interventions when colleagues' behaviors raise concerns. This extremely sensitive position must be handled with care to avoid ruining the career of a colleague. Behavior suspicious for addiction may have many causes and these professionals learn to avoid using the term *addiction* without clear support of such a diagnosis.

Dan, formerly a resident in anesthesiology at a hospital in the Pacific Northwest, spoke with me when he was an inpatient receiving treatment for addiction to fentanyl. "At our hospital we have to check out the drugs from the pharmacy directly, so at the beginning of the day you figure out what you need for the day's cases and then return what you don't use at the end of the day. I returned syringes of saline labeled as fentanyl and kept the fentanyl for myself. Actually, most of the time I had already used it during the day, so there was nothing left to return anyway, but I didn't feel right about charting it as given to a patient, so I just pretended it was leftover." The incongruence between Dan's acceptance of working as a resident while under the influence of fentanyl and having a moral issue with falsifying medical records didn't seem to bother him. "I made sure that my patients got enough fentanyl so they weren't in pain, but after a few weeks I needed so much for myself that I was returning five or six syringes of saline at the end of the day. I guess they got suspicious and actually tested the liquid." Dan felt that he was identified sooner than he would have been had he attributed the diverted fentanyl to patient administration and charted it on the operative reports, but it would likely have been only a matter of weeks. "The reality was that I had had enough. It had been three months at that point and I was miserable. I couldn't stop using on my own, but I was too afraid to ask for help."

Dan was lucky enough to be a resident at a program with a well-established physician wellness committee. The residency program director and committee members all had experience conducting interventions and knew what to do. "The next morning when I came in to work, I got a page from my program director saying that I needed to come by his office. I had never received such a page from him before, so I guessed what was going on." When Dan arrived for the meeting, there were four other people in attendance: the residency program director, the chair of the department of anesthesiology, a trained interventionist and, most surprising to him, his wife. "I recognized everyone there. I couldn't believe they had called my wife too. I had spent the last three months trying to keep this a secret from everyone. I had no idea something like this would ever happen to me."

When conducting an intervention, it is generally better to have a larger group than a smaller one and it is appropriate to include anyone who is close to the individual as long as they are supportive of the intervention and not disruptive. In this case, the individual's spouse was asked to come in and Dan was not paged until his wife had been told the nature of the meeting and agreed to be supportive. Sometimes other family members, friends and colleagues who have witnessed the individual's behavior are asked to participate as well. It is appropriate to include a mixed gender group, especially if the addict is a female. To have an intervention team consisting of all males when the individual is a female can further increase the addict's defenses.

"They confronted me as soon as I sat down and asked me to explain what was going on. When I denied that I had been using, they didn't waste any time." They presented Dan with the evidence suggesting that he had been diverting fentanyl intended for patients from the hospital pharmacy and asked him to provide a urine sample for drug screening. "I actually thought there was a possibility that the test would come up clean and if I just kept denying that I had been using then I would be able to get away and take care of this on my own." When it was clear that Dan would not admit to using drugs, the interventionist tried another approach. "She suggested that maybe I had been diverting the fentanyl to sell on the street. She told me that it was a felony to divert controlled substances from hospital supplies and that if the DEA got involved and I couldn't prove that I had been using and not selling, I would probably do some jail time."

Threats such as this should be used only as a last resort, but when all else fails, threats to involve the authorities coupled with an offer to provide treatment can cause an addict to admit that he or she has a serious problem. "My program director gave me one last chance to admit that I had a problem and get into treatment and I took it." When someone is actively using and addicted, he or she protects him or herself with a wall of denial. An intervention can either build the wall higher or break it down, which is why it is so important that it be done properly.

Dan was not allowed to leave the intervention by himself and he was not allowed to drive. Impaired individuals such as Dan have become suicidal once the gravity of the situation they are in becomes apparent. These people may have a "stash" in their cars or lockers. Prior to the intervention, arrangements are made for direct transfer to an inpatient facility and in this case, a car was waiting to transport Dan once the intervention was conducted. Dan was not allowed to decide what type of treatment he needed. "I was shocked that they wanted me to leave right from the hospital. I didn't even have a toothbrush, but they wouldn't let me go home to get one. I really thought I would just need some time off from work so I could go to an outpatient treatment center, but I had no idea what I really needed. I was so sick that I minimized the extent of my problem."

The considerable tension involved with the process of intervention can be avoided by having an addicted healthcare professional evaluated by a facility off-site from the practice location. Many of the centers designed to assist with the diagnosis and treatment of addictive disorders in this population accept referrals for three- or five-day evaluations. During this period, the addicted healthcare professional is subject to a multidisciplinary evaluation conducted in a partial hospitalization or inpatient setting where he or she can be observed continuously. The individual is interviewed by an addiction medicine physician and an addiction psychiatrist. Psychological and neuropsychological testing is conducted. Additional collateral information is collected from coworkers, family members and other sources and all data is considered by the evaluation team prior to making a recommendation. While there is no data regarding the percentage of individuals referred for this type of evaluation who remain in treatment after their evaluations or who are referred for treatment at different facilities, the frequency is high. This fact is not lost on the inpatient population who often smirk when a newcomer says he or she is "only here for an evaluation." In fact, one facility offers ironic tee-shirts for sale with the slogan "I'm only here for a three-day evaluation" on them.

Improper Confrontation

All too often, instead of proper and safe interventions, addicts are confronted inappropriately. They may be asked to give urine for a drug screening under penalty of termination if they refuse. They may be cornered and abruptly questioned about their unusual use of narcotics, instead of being presented with organized and irrefutable evidence in an atmosphere of care and concern. Worse still, they may be forcibly removed from the hospital by security without any plan in place for detoxification and treatment.

Robert, an attending anesthesiologist at a hospital, described how he "took care" of a known addict whom he was convinced had relapsed. "This resident had been out of work for almost two years, because he had a problem with drugs. For some reason the department let him come back to work and he was part of my call team one night. We have cameras in the operating rooms and I was sitting at the control desk working on the schedule for the next day when I noticed someone walking into an empty room. I had been suspicious of him for some time, so I really wasn't surprised when I saw him taking supplies to inject drugs out of a cart in an empty operating room. When I realized who it was and what he was doing, I called security. We were waiting for him when he came out of the bathroom, where he had just used. I told him we knew what he was doing and that his continued employment in this program was doubtful. Then I asked security to throw him out. I have no tolerance for this sort of behavior on my watch." When I asked if he knew what had ultimately happened to this person, Robert said he had no idea. "He could be dead for all I know; he never came back."

Other members of Robert's department, however, did know what eventually became of this resident. He had been reported to the state board of medicine when he first entered treatment for addiction and had been able to obtain only a provisional license. This relapse was considered a violation of the terms of his probation and his license was revoked. He chose to leave the practice of medicine altogether and had to find employment in another area unrelated to medicine. In retrospect, this choice was probably a wise one for him, as some time after this incident a friend of his who also worked at the same hospital was dismissed for fentanyl diversion, fentanyl that he claimed he was diverting not for his own personal use but to give to this former resident.

The Intern's Affair with Fentanyl

Withdrawal is often difficult and unpleasant, so avoidance of this experience may be the primary reason an addict continues to use in spite of significant negative consequences. Alex, an intern, began using fentanyl as a medical resident. "We had a number of patients with terminal cancer on the palliative care service who had these patches designed to deliver a steady dose of fentanyl over a period of seventy-two hours. If you think about it, someone receiving a dose of 100 micrograms has a patch of 7200 micrograms of fentanyl. That's a lot of fentanyl. I learned from Carol, one of the nurses on the service, that you could open the patch and dissolve the gel to take out the fentanyl. We started using together. I got the patches from the pharmacy or she took them off one of our patients and we went to her place, cooked the gel and then both injected the fentanyl. A few patches yielded a lot, so we only had to take them once or twice a week. It only took about a week before I was hooked."

Alex was married and living with his wife at the time and it wasn't long before she started to notice changes in his behavior. "I started spending a lot more time away from home," Alex explained. "I kept saying that I had to go to work early or stay late but some days I didn't even go in. I went straight to Carol's apartment and got high. The withdrawal each morning was so bad I couldn't do anything without first taking fentanyl. It starts with the realization that you're not high anymore. That warm glow is gone and you start to get restless. For some reason, my ankles itched and I couldn't stop yawning. When that started, I knew it was only a matter of time before things got really bad. If I didn't get my fix, before long I got the sniffles and my eyes started to tear, but the worst was that feeling of cold. I have never been so cold in my entire life. There's nothing you can do to get warm; not even a hot bath helps. Your heart starts to race and you start to ache all over, deep in your bones.

"One weekend I had to stay home, because my wife's family was in town. I spent the whole time vomiting or on the toilet because of diarrhea. It's so hard to go through that knowing that all you need to make everything go away is just one more hit of the drug. It's so easy to say to yourself that you'll just do this one last time and try to kick it the next morning."

Eventually, Alex's wife found out what he had been doing. "The attending physician I was on service with that month called my wife at home when I didn't show up for work two days in a row and my wife got suspicious. When she found out where I was, she assumed I was having an affair with Carol. I guess in some very real way I was having an affair, but not with a woman." Both Alex and Carol were fired from their jobs at the hospital. "They offered each of us a chance to go into a program, but we both refused. I figured my marriage was over and I felt like I couldn't go through the withdrawal, so why bother?"

Alex continued to use whatever he could find for the four months that followed his dismissal from his residency program. "Eventually you reach a point where you'll use whatever you can get just to try to prevent some of the symptoms of withdrawal. Carol got another job at a nursing home. She gave her friend's name and number at the hospital as a reference so her new employer wouldn't find out why she left. We could still get fentanyl every once in a while, but I was taking zolpidem or alprazolam or sometimes even diphenhydramine just to make it through the night. One morning, outside Carol's apartment, I realized my car had been towed. I had no money, no way to get the car back, nowhere to go and that was it. I had just had enough."

Alex called the program director who had dismissed him from his residency program four months earlier and asked for help. He was referred to an inpatient facility which managed his withdrawal through substitution with the long-acting narcotic buprenorphine, with the idea that the drug would be subsequently tapered off while he was still an inpatient. "They told me I was lucky that I had used the day before, because if my admission drug test had not been positive for narcotics then they would not have been able to give me the buprenorphine."

Alternative management of withdrawal during detoxification includes the use of non-narcotic medications like acetaminophen or ibuprofen, but these are much less effective and a fair number of patients terminate the detoxification process prematurely and return to narcotic use. Unfortunately for an addicted healthcare professional who has entered into a contractual agreement with the state healthcare professionals program, early termination of the process results in the revocation of the professional's license to practice.

The Inpatient Experience: What to Expect

Let's look at this from the perspective of an addicted health provider for a moment. Put yourself in the position of an addicted healthcare professional who is ready to enter treatment. Perhaps you have been discovered diverting medications at work, maybe you were just arrested for driving under the influence or maybe you're tired of the addiction. However it happened, your problem came to the attention of the authorities.

Once you have been identified as an impaired healthcare professional who requires treatment for addiction, you will most likely be admitted to an inpatient facility that specializes in the treatment of medical personnel. It is important that such a facility is chosen for a number of reasons. Unlike the standard twenty-eight-day inpatient program that nonmedical personnel often attend, your expected length of stay as a healthcare professional will be considerably longer because of the high risk for individual and patient harm should relapse occur. Intensive inpatient treatment aimed at changing your addictive behaviors may take two or three times as long as is typically allocated for nonmedical personnel. It is not that most addicted persons would not benefit from longer inpatient treatment, but rather that most health insurance plans do not adequately cover the costs of such treatment. Typically, those individuals whose participation is not mandated will not voluntarily partake in such an extended and costly program, but you, as a medical professional, don't have a choice.

If you are going to be allowed to return to clinical practice, then you must be given the best chance to achieve a successful recovery. Typical inpatient lengths of stay for healthcare professionals are eight to twelve weeks, but you may be an inpatient for as long as six to twelve months if the treatment team determines that you are not ready for discharge.

While there are currently no programs in the United States that admit only healthcare professionals, there are about a dozen available that offer programs for physicians and other medical personnel within the larger inpatient population. It is likely that you will find yourself in a facility with considerable expertise in the treatment of addicted healthcare professionals, as some have been providing these services for over three decades.

One such facility is Marworth Alcohol and Chemical Dependency Treatment Center, located in Waverly, Pennsylvania, which offers such a program within a program. "Our healthcare-specific inpatient treatment program typically has about twenty patients at any given time," said Dr. Withers, the program's associate director. "Most of these patients are physicians but can include dentists, vets, nurses and pharmacists. The program is embedded in an overall 12-step oriented program for the public. When we are at full capacity, the total census is about eighty patients."

Many facilities also offer specific programs tailored to the needs of other professional groups such as pilots, firefighters and police officers, so it is likely that you will be interacting with a variety of professionals from different backgrounds. These groups interact with each other during activities that involve the entire population, such as recreational therapy and 12-step study groups, but group therapy sessions are conducted only with the members of the medical professionals program, separated from the general population. Given the sensitive nature of these sessions, there are specific days when the men and women of each group meet separately.

The disease of addiction is one of isolation, especially for addicted healthcare professionals. Since treatment in a facility where the other patients are not physicians or healthcare professionals may lead to an increased sense of isolation and despair or perhaps foster the false belief that you are a special case, you will typically not be the only medical professional in the treatment facility. Seeing oneself as somehow different from the other addicts is often one of the main factors that allowed you to think that you could control your use in the first place. Such a belief is detrimental to recovery. It is important that you see peers in the same situation going through the same treatment and you must develop the support of other similarly affected individuals.

Inpatient treatment typically involves detoxification, monitored abstinence, education, exposure to self-help groups and psychotherapy. Inpatient therapy is typically intensive and you can expect staff contact extending up to twelve hours per day, seven days per week. In this setting, all contact with staff and other patients is potentially therapeutic. You will be removed from the stresses of daily life, as well as from access to alcohol and drugs, and allowed the time you need to focus on your recovery. It can be difficult for someone who has been trained to care for other people to take care of him or herself, but as anyone who has flown in a commercial aircraft is aware, it is essential you place the oxygen mask over your own nose and mouth before attempting to assist other passengers.

Detoxification Essentials

The withdrawal experience depends on the agent on which an addicted health professional has become dependent, but this can be thought of as experiencing the opposite effects of acute intoxication. The period of time it takes for withdrawal to begin depends on the half-life of the drug. The term *half-life* refers to the period of time it takes for half of the drug to be removed from the body, through either metabolism or excretion. If a drug has a half-life of one hour, then one hour after a dose is taken, only 50 percent of that dose remains. That doesn't mean that you will feel half of the effects though, as sometimes only a small amount of the drug is required for its effects to be experienced. The idea of half-life only refers to elimination of the drug from the body.

For most drugs, the entire dose has been removed from the body after five half-lives. For example, if a doctor is experiencing withdrawal from the narcotic fentanyl (which has a very short half-life), he or she will begin to experience a runny nose, watering eyes, muscle and bone aches and shaking chills (among other horrible symptoms) within hours after his or her last injection. If the doctor is taking the narcotic methadone (which has a much longer half-life), he or she may not experience these withdrawal symptoms for days after his or her last dose, but it is likely he or she will experience them for a longer time.

Most addicted healthcare professionals who are identified as possibly having substance abuse problems are immediately sent for evaluation at a program with facilities available for medical monitoring of detoxification. Because withdrawal can sometimes pose significant health risk, it is extremely important that persons who have become physically dependent on any drug go through withdrawal in a monitored setting. While withdrawal from most drugs of abuse is usually not life-threatening, people with coexisting medical conditions or those dependent on alcohol or certain types of drugs are at increased risk of death during this process. The program at Marworth has medical staff available to manage withdrawal and detoxification. "We are able to manage detoxification for most cases, but we refer out patients who are in severe withdrawal from alcohol as these patients are at high risk for death," Dr. Withers explained. Additionally, Marworth accepts patients who have detoxed elsewhere.

Not every healthcare professional goes through detoxification in a monitored setting or even as part of mandated treatment. Charles, a physician, chose to detoxify on his own, but he enlisted the aid of unwitting medical professionals. "I went to the emergency room in the next town over. I lied about who I was and what was going on and got a prescription for clonidine. The three weeks that followed were hell, but the clonidine helped temper the withdrawal somewhat." Charles's experience is typical of an addicted healthcare professional who chooses to go through withdrawal on his or her own. Often, this is a last-ditch effort to avoid treatment but, in most cases, the authorities have already been notified and the investigations have begun. Charles was contacted shortly after detoxification and entered an inpatient treatment program as a requirement of his alternative-to-discipline program.

Background Search

Regardless of how you get into treatment, while you are going through the acute phase of withdrawal, your treatment team is typically collecting collateral information about you through interviews with coworkers, hospital employees, friends and family members. It is not uncommon for intensive background searches on all new patients to include both direct interviews with colleagues and acquaintances and Internet inquiries for information available through public sources such as arrest records or license actions from other locations.

It is important to determine the extent to which your addiction has affected your ability to function in the workplace as well as your family relations and social life. The extent to which your colleagues report impaired ability to function at work has implications for your return to work after treatment and your family of origin and current family structure at home has serious implications for your continued recovery and risk for relapse after discharge. This may contribute to problems or support corrective behavior depending on your individual circumstances. By the time you have made it through the acute withdrawal phase, the treatment team may already know a lot about you. Intake questions at this point may simply serve to verify what the investigation has uncovered and your responses will lay the foundation for the weeks ahead. You may be cautioned: "Are you ready to be completely honest with us? Have you told us everything? Are you holding anything back? Be careful how you answer, because we already know the truth."

Individualized Treatment Plan

The primary goal of inpatient treatment is to lay the groundwork for early recovery; achieving abstinence from drugs and alcohol is only the beginning of the process. The first step in the development of an appropriate treatment plan is a comprehensive assessment, which commonly includes:

- Evaluation by an addiction medicine physician to determine what type of addictive disorder the healthcare professional has and to which agents he or she has become addicted.
- Evaluation by an addiction psychiatrist to determine if the healthcare professional has any psychiatric disorders that need to be considered in treatment.

- Thorough medical history and physical exam to determine the existence of any medical consequences of chronic substance abuse as well as an evaluation of any concurrent medical conditions unrelated to substance abuse.
- Psychological testing to determine the presence of any personality disorders or traits which may require an adjustment in treatment or increase the risk for relapse.
- Neuropsychological testing to evaluate the extent of any cognitive deficit.
- Hair and body fluid testing to corroborate the history of abuse as given by the healthcare professional and to determine the honesty of self-reported drug use.
- Spiritual history to evaluate the extent to which past involvement with religious organizations may support or interfere with a 12-step program based in spirituality.

In cases where the level of honesty of self-reported behavior is suspect, a forensic interview with or without a polygraph exam may be conducted. This is especially true in cases where sexual compulsivity or predatory sexual behavior is an issue and with healthcare professionals who may require treatment for special issues related to sexual addiction. Because of the risk for pseudo-addiction in healthcare professionals with histories of chronic pain, evaluation by a pain specialist may help determine a more appropriate treatment plan.

Self-Help Groups as Part of Early Recovery

Various models of individual and group therapy all aim at altering key addictive behaviors, but most experts agree that an abstinence-based model is the most effective for treatment of addicted healthcare professionals. Since the overwhelming evidence points toward abstinence from all mood-altering chemicals, not just alcohol and other drugs of abuse, as having the greatest likelihood for success in the population of healthcare professionals, an early introduction to a 12-step program such as Alcoholics Anonymous (AA) or Narcotics

Anonymous (NA) is key. There are a number of alternative detoxification and treatment programs available to the general public that offer a wide range of treatment philosophies, but all the healthcare-specific programs use the 12-step philosophy as the core around which all other aspects of treatment are centered. Participation in these self-help groups is considered a vital component in therapy, so you can expect an introduction to self-help programs from day one.

Most treatment centers are based on the Minnesota Model, which is derived from the recovery model of Alcoholics Anonymous, and many healthcare professionals who have attended these programs report the single most effective part of treatment was the introduction to AA or NA. Remember we discussed Willie, the nursing instructor who was addicted to hydrocodone? He said: "I took too many pills one night at work and couldn't function. I was confronted at the end of my shift by the nursing manager who clearly knew what was going on. Since I worked in a small rural hospital with no security, I was driven home by the county sheriff. There was no plan for detoxification or treatment; they just let me go. I agreed to go to an inpatient program after an intervention by my pastor and my best friend." Willie was admitted into an inpatient program that did not specialize in treatment for the addicted healthcare professional. "There were two other nurses in my group and I also made some other contacts. I was in inpatient treatment for approximately nine days and then discharged for six weeks of intensive outpatient treatment. I found more support through AA and NA than in that outpatient group. That was probably what made the difference for me. I got a sponsor and did the twelve steps. Just knowing that I wasn't alone helped more than anything else."

The basic idea behind all the 12-step programs is that by sharing the experience of being an alcoholic or an addict with another similarly affected person, the addicted individual can gain the strength to stay clean and sober. First formed in 1935, Alcoholics Anonymous is a fellowship of people who meet regularly to share their experiences, strength and hope so that they may remain sober. Given the success of Alcoholics Anonymous where other attempts at treatment have failed, it is not surprising that recovery groups based on this 12-step model have formed to address specific issues other than alcoholism. Fellowships for persons addicted to narcotics (Narcotics Anonymous), cocaine (Cocaine Anonymous) and gambling (Gamblers Anonymous) provide forums for mutual support based on the shared experience of addiction to similar agents or compulsive actions.

An introduction to these programs is a large part of the inpatient experience and healthcare professionals are expected to attend ninety meetings during the first ninety days of sobriety. The idea behind the "90 in 90" philosophy is that once you develop the habit of attending a meeting once a day you'll continue to do so and be more likely to maintain sobriety after discharge. You can expect to attend a Narcotics or Alcoholics Anonymous meeting every day you are in treatment. Almost all inpatient programs host meetings every day of the week so that addicted healthcare professionals who cannot leave the facility may still attend the required meetings. Moreover, much of the work conducted in the workshops and small group sessions is focused on completing the first three of the twelve steps.

The twelve steps of any mutual help program differ slightly depending on the organization, but the basic idea is the same. The first step is to admit that you have a problem. In the case of AA, the first step reads: "We admitted we were powerless over alcohol—that our lives had become unmanageable." Simple though it sounds, the first step is a difficult one for many addicted people to take, especially addicted healthcare professionals. You belong to a group of people who often deny any symptoms of disease and rarely seek treatment on your own. As a person who is used to providing care to others, it is difficult for you to assume the patient role and relinquish control.

The second step may present a problem for you as well, especially if you are a scientifically minded healthcare provider, because it requires the recognition of some greater power. The second of the twelve steps is the recognition that this greater power can help: "Came to believe that a Power greater than ourselves could restore us to sanity." Alcoholics Anonymous is not a religious program but rather a spiritual one. If you are unable or unwilling to accept the presence of a greater power, the concept of giving your problems over to another to handle may help. As an addicted healthcare professional in treatment, it is this surrender that is essential, as the third step requires: "Made a decision to turn our will and our lives over to the care of God *as we understood Him.*"

The tradition of anonymity is especially important for health-care professionals in treatment for addiction. The treatment team understands that it may be uncomfortable for you to attend AA or NA groups in the community where you practice. In response to this concern, mutual help groups based on the professions of the addicts instead of the agents to which they have become addicted, such as the Caduceus Group for physicians, have formed. Attendance at these groups is often mandated by post-discharge monitoring contracts.

Individual, Group and Family Therapy

Self-disclosure regarding behaviors related to addiction is essential for recovery. If you have no insight into the nature or severity of your illness you will not get better. The violations of the Hippocratic Oath or other similar professional standards which occur during the period of active addiction can produce great feelings of shame or guilt. If you cannot articulate these feelings it is unlikely that you will be able to overcome them. Groups specific to healthcare professionals allow for sharing of behaviors that may have resulted in patient harm in a more understanding environment.

During these group therapy sessions, you can expect to focus on issues related to your past addicted behavior and the feelings generated by both the behavior itself and the recollection of these past events. To hold back, hedge or say what you think the treatment team wants to hear during these sessions will do no good. The point is not to get this over with but to get this done right. Complete honesty is the most effective road to recovery.

All treatment programs focused on addicted healthcare professionals include some element of family therapy, as it has been shown that involving the persons immediately surrounding the addict leads to better outcomes. A brief program providing an overview of the treatment process and what to expect will be provided to your family members or other guests on visiting day. Just as you are moving through your own stages of denial, anger and fear, so will your family members. By redirecting the negative feelings your family may have away from you or, in some cases, away from the treatment program you are in and toward more constructive areas such as supporting your treatment, the prospects for your success can be increased.

Because of the association between chemical dependence and other psychopathology, successful treatment for addiction is less likely when any psychiatric issues you may have are not also addressed. As an addicted healthcare professional under evaluation or in treatment for substance abuse, you can also expect an evaluation for any comorbid psychiatric conditions. An addictionologist, an addiction psychiatrist who focuses on evaluation and treatment of individuals with alcohol, drug or other substance-related disorders and of individuals with dual diagnosis of substance-related and other psychiatric disorders, will perform the initial evaluation and direct your subsequent treatment.

Monitored Abstinence

Despite attempts by staff to prevent the introduction of drugs or alcohol into the inpatient setting, there will be opportunities for you to obtain your drug of choice. Most treatment centers sponsor Alcoholics or Narcotics Anonymous meetings that are open to inpatients as well as members of the community. Outsiders attending these meetings mingle with inpatients before and after the program. Staff encourage this interaction so that patients in early recovery can make connections in the recovery community outside the institution. It is important for you, with only a few days of sobriety, to see that prolonged recovery is possible and even beneficial. Sadly, it is often during these interactions when drugs exchange hands and more than one person has relapsed while still a patient at an inpatient treatment facility.

Even the strictest of programs allow contact with visitors at some point and you can expect that your family members will be carefully screened prior to visiting. Any suitcases, bags or clothing items that they bring for you will be carefully searched for drugs and alcohol.

Because the potential for relapse always exists, your abstinence is monitored through the use of random urine and breath alcohol checks. In addition to these random checks, facilities with extended inpatient programs that offer long-term patients the privilege of spending weekends at home after reaching a certain point typically collect samples upon returning to the facility.

Chad, a physician assistant who provides medical care for patients at an inpatient treatment facility, revealed a particularly disturbing event that occurred. "The counselors are very specific about not allowing any patient in the healthcare professionals group to provide medical care or advice to the other patients. Their role here is to be a patient, not a provider, and stepping out of the sick role is seen as a roadblock to recovery." All treatment programs with a mixed population have strict limits that prohibit patients in the healthcare professionals group from providing medical advice or treatment to other patients, but sometimes this policy has to be broken. "A lot of the docs here joke about what are they supposed to do if someone has a cardiac arrest—just stand there and wait for me to arrive?" For most of the time, Chad is the only person on site with professional medical training and he is only present during the daytime. The counselors are trained in CPR and automatic defibrillators are available, but at night the reality is that some of the patients have more medical training and experience than the staff. "Last year Lisa, one of the patients, picked up some heroin at an open meeting on campus and overdosed in her bathroom. Lisa fell against the door and her roommate found her right after she went down. The roommate screamed and everyone came running. One of the ER docs and an anesthesiologist, both patients, resuscitated Lisa before the facility staff even got there."

The Cost of Addiction Versus the Cost of Recovery

Inpatient treatment is not inexpensive. Sometime during the second or third week of treatment you may receive a letter from your insurance company explaining that since there is no medical need for you to remain an inpatient, as determined by the doctors at the insurance company, the company will not be paying for the remainder of your mandated treatment.

Cara was a surgical resident before she became addicted to morphine and left the field of medicine for a career in law. "It's been seven years since I was discharged from that inpatient program and I still haven't paid off the credit cards I used to charge my treatment. I remember that second week when they called me into the business office and asked me how I was going to pay for my treatment." Cara's insurance had covered the first two weeks of her stay, but the company refused to pay for any further inpatient treatment. "The insurance company said I could be treated as an outpatient, but the doctors at the treatment center refused to discharge me. They said that I wasn't ready to go and that if I left it would be 'against medical advice.'" If Cara left treatment early, not only would her insurance likely demand repayment for the first two weeks of treatment, but also she would have been reported to the state medical board as noncompliant with the terms of her monitoring.

"It was pretty clear that I didn't have a choice. If I wanted to keep my medical license, I had to come up with the cash to cover the treatment." Cara produced a credit card and authorized the center to charge the $2,900 due. "They asked me to pay a week ahead of time. The wanted me to leave a card on file, but I didn't have one with that kind of a limit on it. By the time I was done I had charged $30,000 on seven different credit cards." Cara was discharged to a halfway house where she spent the six months that followed her initial inpatient treatment. "I was very willful and angry and I suppose it's a good thing that I didn't go back to medicine right away. Those six months at the halfway house gave me a lot of time to think. Even though I was in debt, I decided to go back to school. Ironically, it cost me nine months and the $30,000 I spent trying to save my medical license to figure out that being a surgeon wasn't really the best thing for me."

In addition to the substantial cost of inpatient treatment, you will also have to comply with mandatory urine monitoring schedules once you have been discharged. This must be paid for out-of-pocket as these services are typically not covered by health insurance. This may be difficult if financial issues are present. The cost for collection by an approved monitor and processing of urine or blood samples can be as much as ninety dollars per sample and samples are often collected two or three times per week during early recovery. If you have a history of abusing fentanyl, sufentanil, propofol or any other drug that is not routinely included in the basic screening for drugs of abuse, you can expect the cost per sample to identify these agents to be significantly more.

Susan, who is currently involved with a professional's assistance program and mandated to provide regular urine samples for analysis, must cover a substantial portion of the cost of this monitoring herself. "My insurance covered most of my rehab. I don't remember the amount of my co-pay, but I do remember there was one and it took me a while to pay it off. I now pay $208 per month for urine screenings and $335 every six months for hair screenings and this doesn't include the many thousands of dollars I've already paid and still owe my attorney for defending me in court and for each time I go back to the board." Susan was careful to point out that she does not include the costs associated with her arrest for driving under the influence, a cost related to her addiction but, as she put it, "not associated with recovery."

Evan and Jacob both work for hospitals in the South, both are anesthesia residents in recovery from addiction to fentanyl and both have the same medical insurance. Interestingly, they have had very different experiences with the same company when it comes to getting mandated urine screenings covered. Evan has had far more success. "I've been submitting the bills for the screenings on a monthly basis for reimbursement for the last two years. At first I just sent [the insurance company] the bills that I got from the lab, but they always rejected them, because they didn't have an ordering physician's telephone number or the proper CPT or ICD-9 code on the bill. I called the lab, but really they couldn't be bothered, because they knew I didn't have a choice. They've got a monopoly on the testing for the PHP, so if I want to remain compliant I've got to go with them, and all they care about is whether or not they get paid. So I started modifying the bills using my computer to add all the information they wanted and the insurance company actually started reimbursing me for my out-of-pocket expenses! Every once in a while they reject a claim and I just call repeatedly until they put me in touch with someone who is willing to change the decision in the computer and cut me a check. The people on the other end of the line there don't really know anything about medicine; all they know is numbers and codes, so you have to make sure you give them just enough information so that they can process the claim but not too much so they get confused and deny it."

Jacob's results from submitting the bills for the same services to the same insurance company are the opposite. "Maybe I don't have the time to do what Evan does, but that shouldn't make a difference. It's the same service, it's the same claim and I don't understand why it doesn't get processed the same way." Jacob admitted that he just takes the bill that the lab sends him and forwards it to the insurance company. "When they reject it—and they always do—then I go ahead and pay it. Well, actually I send it to my parents who pay it; I don't actually have any money to pay it myself." Evan expressed contempt for Jacob's lack of motivation. "I don't have the money to pay for this either; that's why I'm so proactive in trying to get these bills covered. The last thing I need is even more debt weighing me down. That's what got me into this mess in the first place. I think Jacob's main problem is that he has no external or internal motivation. His parents need to cut him off."

In this era of cutting costs, it can be tempting to promote less expensive programs for treatment, but as we consider how healthcare will be delivered in this country in the coming years, it is important to remember the costs of untreated addiction are even higher than the costs for addiction treatment. Treatment programs designed for addicted healthcare professionals represent the best choice for addiction treatment. They have proved efficacy far above what is available to the general public; yet because of their costs these programs remain out of reach for most. Even the standard twenty-eight-day programs available to the general public are not fully covered by most health insurance plans and many patients are deemed "ready for discharge" as soon as their insurance stops paying.

The societal costs of addiction are difficult to quantify but include, in addition to money spent on treatment, the opportunity costs of lost productivity, both for the addict as well as the family that has to support him or her. Addiction creates a slow, insidious drain on personal finances and careers and eventually results in ill health and high medical bills. Often, addicts cannot cover these medical costs and they must be absorbed by the rest of society. This increased risk of injury or illness related to addiction and long-term loss of earning capacity due to illness and disability add more stress to what is increasingly becoming an overburdened healthcare system. The costs of crime associated with addiction are considerable. According to the Bureau of Justice Statistics, drug crimes accounted for 18 percent of state prisoners and 51 percent of all federal prisoners in 2009 and 2010 respectively.[4] The costs of raising children whose parent or parents are impaired through addiction must be shouldered by others and this saps resources which could be spent better elsewhere. When all of these direct and indirect costs are compared with the costs for effective treatment, it becomes clear that we could be saving a lot by spending a little more up front for treatment.

Treatment of addicted healthcare professionals involves an extended period of time of which the inpatient portion is only a fraction. You may be tempted to think that you have "completed treatment" at the time you are discharged from your inpatient treatment center, but the majority of the work ahead of you will actually occur in the period after leaving the inpatient setting. As an inpatient, you will attend lectures, small groups and workshops designed to teach you the skills necessary to remain abstinent once you leave the relatively protected environment of the treatment facility. After discharge, you must put these skills into practice in the real world. The post-discharge monitoring and outpatient groups that have been arranged for you extend the safety net and will continue to provide the external motivation to maintain sobriety as you attempt to reenter clinical practice.

CHAPTER 11

Professional Health Programs

Our society invests significant and scarce resources in the education and training of healthcare professionals. When these individuals become impaired through addiction, it is often less expensive in terms of real and human costs to attempt to rehabilitate them instead of removing them from clinical practice. Diversion or alternative-to-discipline programs have been created by state medical and nursing societies and are designed to rehabilitate impaired healthcare professionals and return them to clinical practice. These programs strive to maintain a balance between preservation of these resources (the healthcare providers) and maintenance of patient and public safety.

When a physician, nurse or other healthcare professional is identified as having a substance abuse problem, these programs offer an alternative to the outright suspension or revocation of the license to practice. Provided that the impaired professional complies with the rehabilitation contract, stays in recovery and remains free from the influence of mind- or mood-altering drugs, enrollment in these programs temporarily prevents action by the state licensing board and allows for recovering addicted healthcare professionals' eventual return to clinical practice.

Many people do not favor compassion and treatment over programs which emphasize strict discipline for addicted healthcare professionals. However, I strongly feel that the total cost in terms of human lives (both addicts and patients), human suffering, disorder and inefficiency injected into the healthcare system by addicted healthcare professionals can be reduced considerably by programs which emphasize treatment over punishment. Just as the implementation of drug courts that offer rehabilitation as an alternative to incarceration for individuals convicted of drug-related offenses have successfully lowered recidivism rates and eased the burden on our overcrowded prison system, programs which allow addicted healthcare professionals to enter treatment can reduce costs, increase patient safety and preserve vital human resources.

It has been demonstrated that in areas that have adopted discipline-only models as a way of dealing with impaired nurses, the impaired professionals remain in practice far longer than in locales where alternative-to-discipline options exist. A nurse who works in a discipline-only setting and becomes addicted is acutely aware of the consequences of admitting that he or she has a problem and is much less likely to do so. When accused, the nursing union demands, and rightly so, that due process be followed and it can take months before the impaired practitioner is removed from clinical practice. This scenario plays out similarly when the impaired professional is a doctor or any other healthcare provider.

By allowing impaired healthcare professionals the option of entering a treatment program, the costs associated with investigation and prosecution are eliminated, the potential for patient harm and the costs associated with litigating any resulting malpractice is reduced and the impaired practitioners are more likely to recover successfully and return to practice.

Alternative-to-Discipline Programs for Physicians

In 1958, the Federation of State Medical Boards (FSMB) proposed the need for a system of rehabilitation for physicians found to be impaired by addiction to alcohol or drugs. Despite the recognition that a significant problem existed, little progress was made until 1973 when publication of "The Sick Physician: Impairment by psychiatric disorders, including alcoholism and drug dependence" in the *Journal of the American Medical Association (JAMA)* brought the issue to the forefront.[1] Since the first conference on physician impairment in

1975, the AMA has worked with medical organizations, the government and other interested parties to develop the modern system of physician health programs.

By the summer of 2011, there were physician health programs in forty-five states and the District of Columbia, each sponsored by its respective state medical society. The five states that do not have official diversion programs are in various stages of reorganization and currently monitor impaired physicians directly through each state's medical society. Each state diversion program develops its individual policies regarding treatment contracts and return-to-work procedures independent of the other states and reflects the needs of the population of the state. Though there does exist an umbrella organization, the Federation of State Physician Health Programs (FSPHP), not all state PHPs maintain membership and individual states within the federation have different policies on some issues related to recovery, treatment and monitoring of physician clients.

These PHPs do not provide treatment to impaired physicians but rather serve as independent bodies that supervise and coordinate the process.[2] Since they are not directly involved with the treatment process and hence do not provide the mandated treatment, the perception of a conflict of interest is reduced. Regardless of their structures or origins, these programs provide an essential public service by encouraging early detection of addicted physicians, ultimately removing them from clinical practice sooner than discipline-only programs.

Most states offer an alternative-to-discipline option, commonly under the auspices of the state board of medicine, but the structures of these programs vary from state to state. The majority of these programs are independent nonprofit foundations, while some are a division of a state medical association (35 percent) or a medical board (13 percent).[3] These programs offer addicted physicians the opportunity to enter recovery in supportive environments and allow them to return to clinical practice but only under close supervision. Programs that offer voluntary entry with the opportunity to avoid sanctions on the physicians' medical licenses are more likely to have strong records of success and are associated with earlier entry into treatment and less potential for patient harm. As long as the physicians comply with the stipulations of the programs, any criminal charges or license actions related to their illegal use of drugs are often suspended with the understanding that, should they drop out of the program, they would be subject to prosecution.

The length of post-treatment monitoring contracts is at least five years, during which regular urine and/or hair samples are obtained and examined for evidence of relapse.[4] These contracts specify what continued treatment, such as facilitated group and individual therapy, participation in an anonymous 12-step program, follow-up or aftercare is required, though in most cases this treatment is not provided by the physician health program.

All physician health programs are responsible for tracking the abstinence of the physicians with whom they have monitoring contracts. In theory they use random and witnessed body fluid analysis, though in practice these samples may not always be collected in a random manner or entirely witnessed. Most often the samples collected for analysis are urine, although given the increased recognition that these samples may be faked, some state programs are moving to include hair and blood samples as well. Urine screening for physician addicts in recovery includes a panel of twenty to twenty-five different drugs with abuse potential, but does not include the narcotics fentanyl, alfentanil or sufentanil, which must be added to each screening if an individual has a history of abusing these substances. Body fluid is collected in greater frequency at the beginning of the monitoring contract, with most programs requesting six to eight samples per month for the first year and decreased frequency of collection as the period of clean time increases.

In addition to the common goals of early identification and referral to treatment for physicians with substance abuse issues, physician health programs may also provide addiction education programs for physicians and other healthcare professionals. The content of these educational programs as well as their availability varies and is a reflection of the limited resources available in some areas. Most PHPs operate on a meager $500,000 per year, although there is a wide range in operating budgets with some programs receiving only $20,000 from licensing boards, participant fees, state medical associations or contributions from hospital or malpractice insurance companies. Physician health programs are expected to provide all of the administrative and monitoring services for every program participant and this rarely leaves funding for other services, preventing some programs from adequately fulfilling this part of their mission.

Alternative-to-Discipline Programs for Nurses

Due in part to the success of the physician programs, the American Nurses Association's House of Delegates passed a resolution in 2002 promoting alternative-to-discipline programs submitted by several constituent member associations.[5] Despite these efforts, five states still have entirely disciplinary approaches: Alaska, Arkansas, Georgia, Maine and Mississippi. Iowa, Maine and Missouri have statutes allowing alternative-to-discipline programs, but have no operating alternative-to-discipline programs. The Arkansas board of nursing presented legislation in 2010 that would allow an alternative-to-discipline program. When queried, the Georgia board of nursing responded that it is "looking into programs." Alaska has no agenda for a program and cited the "associated administrative costs" as a primary barrier to implementation.

Both alternative-to-discipline and discipline-only programs have reported success rates of 70 to 90 percent for reentry into clinical practice after initial treatment for addicted nurses.[6] Both types of programs have consistently helped a majority of nurses recovering from addictive disorders to reenter the workforce, but the alternative-to-discipline programs remove impaired nurses from practice in a matter of days or weeks compared with the months or years it takes discipline-only programs to remove addicted nurses from clinical practice. While the end result may seem the same, the carrot offered by the alternative-to-discipline programs protects both the addicted nurses and the public sooner and likely results in less opportunity for patient harm.

The success of a program may also be measured in terms of recovery or retention. Depending on the program, rates of recovery range from 50 to 95 percent and rates of retention for nurses range from

60 to 85 percent, but these success rates reveal little about the progress made nationwide in addressing substance use disorders among healthcare professionals.[7] Given the stigma that is still attached to professionals with substance use disorders, the number of nurses who do not receive adequate treatment is not surprising but is still alarming. Many nurses do not have the opportunity to enter these programs. Possibly their managers do not believe in treatment for addictive disorders and dismiss the addicted nurses instead of referring them to treatment. This is considerably more likely to happen in states with no alternative-to-discipline programs, but nurses who have not been adequately treated may not necessarily stay in these states. It is very common for addicted nurses to move to other states in an attempt to "start over." Without adequate treatment, there is no reason to believe the same abuse process will not begin again somewhere else.

Reentry into the workplace is an important issue for administrators, leaders and the public. The American Association of Nurse Anesthetists (AANA) has traditionally advocated for public safety through the removal and safe return of certified registered nurse anesthetists (CRNAs) suffering from addiction, yet AANA recognizes the precarious nature of this undertaking and maintains high standards for reentry. Reliance upon the respective state board of nursing for treatment referrals, long-term monitoring and appropriate reentry is difficult, largely due to the wide discrepancies and inconsistencies among states. I believe what is needed is a set of clearly defined national standards which maximize both treatment outcomes for affected individuals and patient safety.

Alternative-to-Discipline Programs for Other Healthcare Professionals

Most states have diversion programs available for other types of addicted healthcare professionals as well. One example of such programs is Peer Assistance Services (PAS), a nonprofit program that has provided health assistance services in the state of Colorado for licensed dentists, pharmacists, pharmacy technicians and pharmacy students as well as nurses since 1984. The agency provides multiple programs, including evaluation and treatment referral for healthcare providers with substance abuse, psychiatric and/or physical problems that could impair their practice. Funding for these services is received through license renewal fees, though a fee-for-service structure is in place for addicted healthcare professionals not currently licensed in the state.

The program for impaired pharmacy professionals in Washington, called the Washington Recovery Assistance Program for Pharmacy (WRAPP), describes itself as a program designed to "protect the health and safety of the public" while also effectively functioning as an employee assistance program. As part of this mission, any person who reports information on a suspected impaired practitioner is immune from civil liability, provided the report is made in good faith. As with the Colorado program, the Washington program provides confidential help with referrals for evaluations, treatment placements and medical services. Individuals sign monitoring contracts similar to those required of physicians and nurses and their progress through treatment, aftercare, rehabilitation and reentry into the workplace is closely watched. The Washington State Board of Pharmacy pays for the program and there are no fees for the services, but just like the equivalent physician or nursing programs, any evaluations, treatments or drug screenings that are required must be paid for by the participant. Compliance with the terms of the WRAPP contract ensures anonymity.

Following successful completion of the inpatient treatment program, formerly addicted healthcare professionals are discharged either to a halfway house or directly to the community. Most states allow these healthcare professionals to return to work after inpatient treatment as long as they remain under the supervision of a health and well-being organization, such as those sponsored by the state medical or nursing society. The onus for continued monitoring of the healthcare professional in early recovery transfers from the inpatient facility to one of the state-sponsored alternative-to-discipline programs. The ultimate decision regarding return to work is usually made after considerable discussion involving both parties.

Monitoring Contracts

Healthcare professionals in recovery who wish to maintain their professional statuses are typically required to sign monitoring contracts that include regular contact with caseworkers at the monitoring organization, worksite observation and random urine drug and alcohol screenings for a minimum period of time. These contracts mandate the complete abstinence from all mood-altering drugs, participation in facilitated group psychotherapy with other recovering medical professionals (Caduceus Group meetings) and regular attendance and participation in self-help fellowships such as Alcoholics Anonymous or Narcotics Anonymous.

The actual composition of these return-to-work contracts differs depending on the state and the profession. In New York, nurses have to commit to two years of monitoring once they return to work while physicians have to sign five-year contracts that begin at the time of their initial removal from clinical practice. Often, though, these contracts are extended at the time the physicians return to clinical duties, especially if legal hearings are needed to reinstate the professionals' licenses to practice.

The terms of reinstatement often include a probationary period and require that physicians sign another five-year contract with the starting date the same as the return-to-work date. In the case of a healthcare professional with a coexisting psychiatric illness such as bipolar disorder, the individual may be required to participate in a monitoring program for the remainder of his or her medical career.

Typical monitoring during this period also differs from state to state but always includes frequent urine samples analyzed for signs of relapse. Some states do not recognize the validity of hair samples and do not mandate this type of testing, because insurance will not cover it. Other states mandate hair testing in addition to urine testing and require program participants to pay for this themselves. If a healthcare professional was treated for alcohol-related impairment, breath testing may also be required. Regardless of the terms of the contract, for those healthcare professionals in recovery wishing to return to clinical practice, full disclosure to management, as well as full support from the clinical department, is essential.

It is important to note that monitored recovery or imposed abstinence is not the same as self-guided recovery and does not hold the same prospects for successfully avoiding relapse. Healthcare professionals often enter into these monitoring contracts under considerable duress. These are not voluntary agreements. Frequently the driving factor is healthcare professionals' desire to maintain the ability to practice and not necessarily the desire to remain sober.

The ever-present threat of loss of livelihood should a drug screening return positive is a strong motivational factor for not using drugs, but this is not recovery. The disease of addiction is suppressed by the commitment to abstinence but only as long as the behavioral and urine monitoring continues. Treatment during this period is intended to shift the drive to maintain sobriety from an external source to an internalized state of self-motivated recovery.

Relapse in a Monitoring Program

The disease of addiction is characterized by chronic, relapsing course. Since there are significant consequences for both healthcare professionals who relapse as well as for the patients they care for, monitoring programs have developed a system of relapse management designed to mitigate risk and reduce the potential for harm. Recognizing that relapse begins with behavioral changes, such as skipping required mutual-assistance meetings, missing therapy appointments or lying about certain aspects of recovery, and ends when the addict actually begins to use drugs again, different levels of relapse with differing levels of response have been identified.

It is not uncommon for healthcare professionals to exhibit relapse behavior or experience an actual "slip" and use drugs again during the first year of recovery. If managed properly, this relapse does not necessarily result in treatment failure or necessitate readmission to an inpatient facility, as long as patient harm has not occurred.

Behaviors such as not showing up for scheduled group therapy meetings or individual therapy appointments and either lying about attending mutual help meetings or refusing to go altogether are suggestive of early relapse. These infractions are typically dealt with by the case manager in the monitoring program as soon as they occur rather than allowing these behaviors to persist; to do so may send the message that monitoring is somewhat more lax than it should be.

If a recovering healthcare professional is discovered to be using drugs or alcohol outside of the workplace, this behavior represents a more serious level of relapse and requires a more aggressive intervention by the monitoring team. Since the healthcare professional is again using drugs, he or she is typically removed from clinical practice until a full evaluation can be performed. Often, a full reassessment of the healthcare professional's commitment to recovery as well as the strength of the family and social support system is required and recommendations may include lengthening the monitoring contract, including more frequent testing and the addition of medications such as naloxone. Should a healthcare professional experience a relapse within the context of the clinical setting, such as while on call or actually at work, the licensing board is almost always notified and a return to inpatient treatment is mandated. All of these measures are undertaken by the professional health programs to protect the individual healthcare professional as well as prevent harm to the public.

Narcotic Maintenance Therapy

For physicians who wish to return to clinical practice while on narcotic replacement therapy with methadone or buprenorphine, the majority of state-sponsored physician health programs do not have official policies either in support of or disallowing the practice. Only ten states explicitly do not allow physicians to return to clinical practice while on narcotic maintenance, with the remainder allowing the practice only in certain situations. States that allow physicians to return to clinical practice while maintained on buprenorphine typically report either evaluating each case on its own merits or having a policy of leaving all treatment decisions to the treatment team and monitoring physicians in recovery without making recommendations.

States that do not support the use of narcotic maintenance typically cite very high abstinence success rates and report concerns with cognitive impairment, stating that this is problematic and would preclude return to work in most cases. Most of these programs have adopted the policy of evaluating each participant on an individual basis to determine how appropriate it would be for someone to return to practice if there has been an interruption, including those individuals who have been placed on buprenorphine maintenance. However, slow discontinuation of the buprenorphine is recommended prior to reentry. In cases where discontinuation of narcotic maintenance presents too great a risk for relapse, the recommendation is not to return to the practice of clinical medicine.

The state physician health programs that do allow physicians to return to work while on narcotic maintenance also cite evidence that abstinence models of treatment and monitoring are the most successful, although despite this, they take the stance that in some cases there is no alternative. These programs have cited concerns with disallowing what may in some cases be a lifesaving treatment. The physicians who are allowed to work while on buprenorphine or methadone have reportedly been on stable doses for a long time (months to years) and have undergone a full battery of neuropsychiatric testing prior to returning to clinical practice to make sure there are no significant cognitive problems that would impair their ability to practice safely.

These programs report being very conservative when monitoring anesthesiologists and other high-risk medical specialties, because they have easy access to highly addictive drugs such as fentanyl and propofol and can become immediately impaired in the workplace. One state which allows physicians to return to clinical practice while on narcotic therapy specifically does not allow anesthesiologists to do so and reports that it will not allow the practice until studies demonstrate a rate of relapse less or equal to those who are completely abstinent. As well, there is debate about whether or not anesthesiologists should ever return to operating rooms, considering the risk of accidental overdose, death or patient injury should a relapse occur.

The few state physician health programs that do not report involvement in treatment decisions emphasize that they were specifically tasked with monitoring the treatment and continuing care of regulated health professionals with illnesses that, if left untreated, might affect their ability to practice safely. As such, they do not provide treatment and decisions such as the use of methadone or buprenorphine are left to the discretion of the individual treatment providers. If narcotic maintenance therapy is recommended, then the treatment is allowed and cognitive testing specific for physicians is conducted at the recommendation of the addictionologist when return to clinical practice becomes possible. While none of the physician health program representatives I contacted would release specific numbers, each indicated that the percentage of physicians currently on buprenorphine maintenance therapy comprises a very small percentage of the overall population of monitored physicians.

When inquiring about individual state policy regarding the use of buprenorphine and reentry for nurses in recovery from addiction, representatives in several states said that it was up to the discretion of the treating addictionologist or counselor. Some state administrators I contacted were adamantly opposed to the use of buprenorphine or methadone, while others allowed all levels of nurses to reenter on it. Then there are those states that either have no policy regarding return to work on these medications or refused to disclose the details of their policies altogether. Much like the physician alternative-to-discipline programs, there is little agreement among the nursing programs in different states.

There is also the issue of compliance. As we saw in the story of Michelle, an addicted nurse, a common characteristic of the drug addict is oppositional defiance, which must be broken down during the recovery process. When a recovering healthcare professional is given a prescription for buprenorphine, he or she might feel that he or she is obliged to take it without question in order to remain in good graces with the monitoring program. The fact that organizations such as AANA do not endorse narcotic maintenance therapy for nurses who wish to return to clinical practice further confuses the matter. It is clear, in my opinion, that the time for a national policy on this issue has come.

Alternative-to-discipline programs serve to advocate for the practitioners, their families, their employers and the licensing boards to support recovery and facilitate safe return to work. They have proven records of success and are essential parts of comprehensive policies designed to deal with the problem of addicted healthcare professionals. These programs play a significant part in the successful rehabilitation of healthcare professionals in recovery who wish to return to clinical practice.

CHAPTER 12

Recovery and Prospects for Returning to Work

W hether healthcare professionals should be allowed to return to clinical practice after being discharged from inpatient treatment remains highly controversial. Addiction is a chronic, relapsing disease with no cure and many believe it is not worth the risk of harm to patients (and practitioners) inherent with returning a professional with a known history of addiction to such safety-sensitive positions. I personally believe that every case should be examined on its own merits and that to embrace a "one strike, you're out" policy is both short-sighted and reactionary.

Historically, a distinction was made between the type of healthcare professional and the level of training he or she had completed prior to being removed from clinical practice for substance abuse. The premise was that an attending physician or established nurse has fewer career options and should be given a chance to reenter practice while a resident or medical student should be encouraged to find another field or specialty. Decisions based on what is perceived as "easier" for an impaired professional do not take into account what is best for both the professional and for our society as a whole. Additionally, there is some speculation that medical specialties such as anesthesiology or emergency medicine represent much greater risks for relapse than other specialties and that healthcare professionals with substance abuse issues should be encouraged to choose "less risky" specialties.

There is little known about what happens once professionals have retrained in different specialties. We also do not currently know what happens to those healthcare professionals who are encouraged to retrain in other fields or even to leave medicine or nursing altogether. Are other specialties really less risky or are we just shifting the problem to another area for someone else to deal with? Provided an individual has been deemed an acceptable risk for return to clinical practice, I believe it would be more prudent for the addicted individual to remain within sight of an effective monitoring program in a field or specialty with a deeper understanding of addiction and the reality of relapse.

Recovery takes time to establish and treatment cannot be rushed. Too often an attending physician who has successfully completed a short course of inpatient treatment is asked to return to work full-time in the same stressful practice without any period allowed for recovery work. The result is often disastrous. Residency programs and medical schools, however, are better able to absorb a part-time healthcare professional in early recovery and provide the slow reentry into clinical practice that may allow motivated individuals to pursue careers in medicine. I strongly feel the decision to allow an individual to return to medical practice should be made on a case-by-case basis, regardless of the type of profession, area of specialty or level of training.

What the Experts Say About Returning to Work

Fred, a case manager with several years' experience treating impaired healthcare professionals in New York State, told me, "In New York, the nurses fall under the Office of the Professions and their Professional Assistance Program (PAP) and the physicians are governed by the Committee on Physician Health (CPH). The program for nurses is wonderful. They get assigned a case manager who tracks them the whole way through the length of their contract and who is a huge advocate for the nurse's success in recovery. The Committee on Physician Health tends to be less involved and somewhat less caring toward the docs and it's also a private organization and not part of the state, so maybe that has something to do with it."

When I asked whether or not recovering healthcare professionals should be allowed to return to clinical practice, Fred echoed the sentiments of most in his field: "I think once there is a solid base in recovery they should be able to go back to work. Would you deny diabetics the right to support themselves if they spike or drop [their glucose levels] and need care?" The comparison that Fred drew between the disease of addiction and diabetes makes the point that both are medical issues for which there are no cures and which require regular maintenance therapy. Both conditions have the potential to harm both the individual with the disease and his or her patients if not properly controlled, but Fred recognized that we currently do not (typically) enroll diabetic healthcare professionals in monitoring programs to make sure they keep their glucose under control. He added, "There should be some degree of supervision and monitoring on the worksite when the addict in recovery returns to work."

For nurses in New York, direct return to work is not allowed immediately upon discharge from an inpatient facility. This makes more sense than what can happen to other healthcare professionals in early recovery. Typically, a nurse must complete an aftercare program as well, which consists of six to twelve months of intensive outpatient treatment. Once the treatment team has determined that it is safe to allow the nurse in recovery to return to clinical work, a personalized contract is drawn up that may have limits on work hours and access to narcotics, depending on the specifics of the case. This delayed return to clinical practice has been shown to be an effective method for managing anesthesia residents who wish to return to residency training in anesthesiology and is the method that I propose should be the national standard.

A member of the treatment team at a facility which provides services for nurses in recovery is also in favor of such an approach. "These professionals should not be allowed to return to work without aftercare and monitoring. The inpatient environment is a safe but artificial and tightly controlled environment. Sobriety must be established in the community where these people live and presumably with the same level of access to the drugs and alcohol they abused before. If they can't stay sober in this environment, then they certainly won't be able to when they return to work." When I asked if these people should be asked to retrain in a "less risky" field, the case worker replied, "Not unless their profession is a whisky taster or drug sampler. The profession is a factor in use but not the deciding factor. Going to work did not make the person take drugs."

There is a high likelihood that physicians in training in any given academic residency program will have to deal with the issue of resident substance abuse.[1] The frequency with which this issue arises depends upon the size of the program and the number of residents in each class, but even the smaller programs will have an addicted resident at some point. Despite the standards regarding the types of cases a resident has to perform or particular diseases a resident has to manage during the course of training to ensure that all physicians graduate with a similar level of experience and skill, there are no guidelines regarding what should be done when a resident becomes impaired through addiction to drugs or alcohol.

Decisions regarding treatment, dismissal from the program or retraining are often made on a case-by-case basis and based on the varied experience and knowledge of the residency program director.[2] When considering whether or not to allow a resident to return to work after treatment, access to the former drug of choice is certainly relevant.[3]

Historically, fentanyl has been the most common drug of choice among healthcare professionals who are addicted to narcotics due to its availability and a pharmacokinetic profile that allows the user to continue to function while at work, albeit at a significantly reduced capacity. Should a resident with such a history of addiction be allowed to return to work in an environment with access to this drug? Recognizing the high abuse liability of this and other major narcotic medications, hospital pharmacies have placed stricter controls on intravenous narcotics and decreased availability of these agents. Relevant questions which should be addressed include: Is it possible that this reduced availability may allow the safe return to clinical practice for residents formerly addicted to these medications or is the increased incidence in abuse of oral agents obtained from outside sources a reflection of the continued desire for these types of drugs?

Relapse After Returning to Work

As much as 25 percent of healthcare professionals will relapse at least once during their first five years of recovery and most of these relapses occur during the first year after initial treatment.[4] Does it make sense to allow a healthcare professional who was formerly addicted to return to clinical work in this environment where easy access to his former drug of choice seems to invite a relapse?

In an attempt to identify factors which may be associated with an increased risk for relapse and hopefully avoid placing recovering individuals in unsafe positions, some investigators have looked closely at what recovering healthcare professionals who were unable to maintain sobriety have in common. Most had family histories of substance abuse, had been using fentanyl or some other major narcotic or had been diagnosed with a psychiatric disorder such as depression, anxiety or bipolar disorder. Individuals who had two or more of these factors were found to be significantly more likely to experience a relapse. When considering whether or not to allow a particular healthcare professional to return to work in his or her chosen field, access to addictive medications is not the only factor to consider.

There seems to be no consistent way in which the issue of re-entry into the clinical workplace is handled across different states, institutions in the same state and, in some instances, even within the same institution. There is no doubt that this is an emotional issue that stirs up strong feelings in those who are involved and these feelings may play a considerable role in decisions that have very real effects on people's lives.

Andy, the residency program director for an anesthesiology residency, stated, "No one wants to make a decision that may end up getting someone killed. We try to avoid that on a daily basis in the operating room. Why would anyone in their right mind allow an anesthesiologist who was addicted to fentanyl to return to clinical anesthesia? It would be like handing them a gun and saying, 'You know what to do with this.' There's no way I could live with myself if something were to happen." Andy has personal experience with resident physicians returning to work after treatment. "I've seen a few people do it successfully but most don't, and when they relapse there's a good chance they're going to die."

Two years ago, a resident who had successfully completed a rehabilitation program and was in a monitoring program at the hospital where Andy is employed was found to be using drugs again. "This guy had eighteen months of clean time, or at least I thought he did. Who really knows, I guess. If he hadn't been caught by one of my colleagues he might be dead. He's not practicing medicine anymore, but at least he's alive." When I asked about what he'll do the next time this issue comes up, Andy replied "I can't do it anymore. We now have a 'one strike, you're out' policy."

Strong emotions such as the ones Andy and other program directors like him express require a clearly defined plan of action based on evidence and experience. While we have plenty of experience, we do not currently have the evidence to point to and say "this is what we should do." Unfortunately, this problem does not lend itself to such a simple solution. Despite the lack of strong evidence to suggest that one protocol works better than another when a healthcare professional in recovery wishes to return to work, there are many opinions on the subject.

Jake, the chairperson of a department at an academic teaching hospital in California, revealed, "I favor allowing a resident or medical student to return to work after treatment, but I would only take them back on the recommendation of the treating physician or psychiatrist and only if they are maintained under strict observation with frequent mandatory urine or hair testing." In addition to experience with residents, Jake reported having to address this issue with some of his colleagues as well. "During the last ten years, two (out of a total of seventy positions) of our faculty members have also had problems. One was dismissed after relapse; the other also relapsed but continues to work. Neither was allowed resident supervision or contact."

Each of these individuals was allowed to return to work with monitoring and mandated Narcotics Anonymous or other self-help group sessions and individual therapy, but given the high relapse rates and the initial presentation of relapse as death, I wonder if treatment for this disease has improved. A question which looms and needs further research is: Is the drug culture too prevalent in generation X, generation Y and the boomers and if so, why?

Environmental Cues in the Workplace

When a healthcare professional in recovery eventually returns to clinical practice, he or she will ultimately find him or herself back in the same environment in which he or she formerly used drugs. Environmental cues as subtle as the smell of the antiseptic solution used to clean the bathroom where the provider self-administered injectable medications can trigger intense cravings and produce an involuntary physiological response which could ultimately lead to relapse.[5] First proposed by Abraham Wikler, the "conditioned withdrawal" model for relapse has its roots in classic Pavlovian conditioning theory. This cue-induced craving and reactivity is thought to be a conditioned response in which exposure to certain stimuli can elicit a very real physiological response in formerly addicted individuals.

When formerly addicted healthcare professionals who have returned to clinical practice are asked to describe the cues they experienced upon their return, they provide a wide variety of responses. Many report cue reactivity related to the hospital bathroom. Being offered a bathroom break or, once inside the room, the smell of the bathroom cleaner have been reported as producing intense cravings in some individuals, presumably since this is where many healthcare professionals formerly self-medicated in isolation. Other cues include the smell of alcohol wipes, the feel of a syringe, the action of drawing up medications and the sight of the ampule containing the drug of choice. Physiological responses such as changes in skin temperature, skin conductance level or heart rate are measurable immediately after exposure and are strongly coupled with subjective responses such as self-reported intensity of cravings or feelings of withdrawal sickness.

The cue literature is extensive, with many instruments already having proven reliability and validity in the evaluation of these unconscious responses. Despite this, experts agree that very little is known about this phenomenon in recovering healthcare professionals, let alone the implications or utility as part of a comprehensive program of reentry. I feel that if a healthcare professional is to return to work in the same environment, he or she should be exposed and desensitized to potential cues in a controlled and supervised environment, but there is little experience with extinguishing responses in this population. A healthcare professional who wishes to return to clinical practice is at high risk for relapse, but it is possible that by reducing or eliminating the physiological response to environmental cues, the risk for relapse can be reduced.

Abstinence is only the beginning of recovery. Maintaining sobriety in recovery from substance abuse is an extremely important and sometimes difficult task. For our purposes, formerly addicted healthcare professionals are considered to be in recovery as long as they are no longer self-medicating with alcohol or illicit drugs and are making a concerted effort to become productive members of society. This also includes the development of effective coping skills and the ability to find pleasure in activities that do not involve the use of recreational pharmaceuticals. For the former addict who is in early recovery, abstinence can be a very tenuous thing.

Addictionologists recommend staying away from the people, places and things associated with using drugs and forming new associations with other members of the sober community. For a formerly addicted healthcare professional who goes back to work, this can be almost impossible. A physician who used to shoot fentanyl in the hospital bathroom will inevitably find him or herself in the same bathroom at some point and will need to deal with the cravings induced by subtle cues, such as the odor of the bathroom sanitizer or the sound of the door latch. Just like Pavlov's dogs, who were conditioned to salivate at the ring of a bell, smells and sounds formerly associated with drug use trigger intense drug cravings which arise from the subconscious. It is extremely difficult to maintain sobriety in this situation without strong coping skills and an effective sober support system, which is why addicted healthcare professionals typically spend much more time as inpatients prior to discharge and why outpatient therapy is mandated during the first year of recovery.

Some addicts are unable to remain clean without the use of opioid replacement therapy (ORT) and may need to take medications,

such as methadone or buprenorphine, that help avoid relapse by preventing the user from experiencing the high associated with narcotic
abuse. Many experts believe ORT is not true recovery since it is not
abstinence-based sobriety and may distinguish between the patient
in a drug-free recovery program and the patient on maintenance
medication. For many healthcare professionals in early recovery who
find themselves in a monitoring program, this intense observation
provides the safety net that helps them avoid relapse.

Robin, a physician assistant, has been in recovery for three years.
"There comes a point when compliance with the program becomes
true abstinence and sobriety, but that very rarely happens during
the first year. As a group, we are highly motivated people, very well
practiced in the art of delayed gratification. For most in the medical
area, becoming licensed medical professionals involved late nights
studying in the library while our friends were out partying, extended
periods of training with long hours and low pay while our same-age
contemporaries were developing careers and some were making large
amounts of money in the early years after college. If we want to, we
can wait for just about anything. The monitoring program kept me
sober until I truly wanted to be. If the program wasn't in place, then
I definitely would have relapsed; I see that now."

Not every healthcare professional in early recovery is as motivated as Robin. Greg, the risk-taking rheumatologist whom we discussed earlier, had already relapsed once when I spoke to him during
his second admission to an inpatient treatment facility. Despite having
completed an eight-week inpatient program and participating in a
post-discharge monitoring program, he was still unable to remain
clean. "These programs are designed to keep you clean until you
actually want to be, but they only work if they're run properly." Greg
knew the person who monitored his urine personally. "I showed
up on the same day each week under the guise that this was for
his convenience and dropped off a clean urine sample. He never
once actually watched me urinate and by the end of my last run I
brought clean urine that wasn't even mine." It also didn't hurt that
his monitor, another physician in his multispecialty group, had a
financial incentive to keep the only rheumatologist they had gain-
fully employed.

As it turns out, Greg never actually stopped using, even during his second admission. He was somehow able to bring a supply of hydrocodone into the treatment facility and continued to take the pills without being detected. When he was granted special privileges after several weeks as an inpatient and was allowed to leave the treatment facility for short periods of time, his first stop was the closest pharmacy where he attempted to fill a prescription for his drug of choice. The addiction professionals at the treatment center must have known something wasn't quite right with him as eventually he was discovered. Greg was transferred to a secondary facility with experience treating more difficult cases where he spent twelve months in a sober community trying to learn how to live without the influence of mind-altering medications.

Relapse is considered part of the disease of addiction and it is expected that a significant number of healthcare professionals in recovery will experience one or more relapses during the course of their treatments. Rather than focusing on relapse as the failure of treatment, it is important to define relapse in terms that allow for early identification and intervention. Addicts relapse long before they pick up drugs and start reusing. It is the return to the thoughts and behaviors which allowed addicts to rationalize their previous drug use that marks the beginning of this relapsing process. If the changes in personality and behavior which herald relapse are recognized, either by the addict or by close friends and family, the relapse process can be interrupted and the eventual return to drug use prevented.

Avoiding Triggering Agents

All mood-altering substances, even those that are medically indicated, have the potential to trigger a relapse. In addition to avoiding the persons, places and things that can provoke drug cravings, avoidance of any potential triggering agents is an essential part of recovery from substance abuse. Unfortunately there are some situations in which avoidance of these agents is impossible. It is very likely that healthcare professionals in recovery will be faced with the dilemma of what to do when exposure to potential triggering agents is inescapable. Formerly addicted healthcare professionals who need surgery or procedures requiring anesthesia are in unique situations, as the mood-altering substances to which they will be exposed are quite frequently the drugs to which they were formerly addicted. Given the high stakes associated with relapse in this population, great care is necessary when healthcare professionals in recovery are exposed.

A number of different techniques can be employed to avoid the use of narcotics and other potentially addictive agents or to help prevent relapse in susceptible individuals if use of these agents cannot be avoided. Nonconventional methods such as hypnosis, guided imagery, acupuncture, meditation, biofeedback, electrical stimulation, transcutaneous electrical nerve stimulation (TENS) and physical therapy, as well as more common methods for treating milder pain such as rest, cold, heat and elevation, have proved to be fairly successful.

Therapies that involve mind over body techniques can be very effective in the treatment of pain resulting from various medical conditions, including postsurgical and chronic pain, but Western medicine has not moved beyond the biomedical model to a biopsychosocial model for several reasons. Despite long records of successful use (many of these treatments have been around for thousands of years and continue to be commonly used in other parts of the world), these alternative treatments are often overlooked, frequently underutilized and not part of the curriculum in most Western medical education programs.

When Exposure Can't Be Avoided

Despite the need to prevent exposure to triggering agents, sometimes exposure can't be avoided. In this situation, well-developed distress tolerance skills can make the difference between relapse and sobriety. The first line of defense should be for healthcare professionals in recovery to attend a 12-step meeting and to call their sponsors or someone else in the program. If their sponsors are not immediately available or it is not possible to attend a meeting, there are other things that can be done to avoid a relapse. Suggestions of things to do to in the face of considerable distress to lessen its impact include:

- Engaging in activities that distract you from the impulse to use or from the stress of the crisis, such as exercising, participating in a hobby, cleaning, going to an event, taking a walk, playing a computer game, balancing your checkbook, gardening or anything that will take your mind off using drugs.
- Contributing to someone or an organization by doing volunteer work, donating supplies or materials to someone else, participating in random acts of kindness or doing a thoughtful act for someone else.
- Making a gratitude list to appreciate all the good things, people and opportunities in your life.
- Partaking in events or activities that create different emotions such as reading a joke book, watching a funny movie or listening to inspiring music.
- Pushing away the situation by leaving it for a while. Build imaginary walls around yourself and the situation, put the pain in a box and place it on a shelf; block it out of your mind for a while.
- Applying other thought methods such as counting to ten, counting colors in a painting or nature or reading 12-step literature.
- Focusing on other sensations such as holding a piece of ice in your hand until it melts, squeezing a rubber ball very hard, standing under a hot shower or snapping a rubber band on your wrist.

Things that can be done to "improve the moment" during particularly stressful periods include using imagery, prayer or relaxation techniques. Guided imagery involves imagining relaxing scenes such as a secret room within yourself that is a safe place. You can go to the room when you feel threatened and imagine the hurtful emotions draining out of you like water out of a pipe. Sometimes it helps to find or create meaning in the pain and understand that there are no coincidences. Eventually, the pain and longing of addiction become easier to deal with. It may also help to have a firm belief in a higher power and, if you do, to ask for strength to tolerate the moment. If all else fails, you can take a brief vacation from everything.

Full Disclosure

It is essential that healthcare professionals in recovery make the treatment teams caring for them aware of the potential for relapse after exposure to addictive agents, but the stigma of being an addict is a harsh reality. Despite considerable education and training, many healthcare professionals with no personal experience with addiction can be judgmental and intolerant of drug addicts. Often, these people view addiction as a weakness or a moral issue and not as a disease that requires treatment just like diabetes or asthma. It is not surprising that addicts are reluctant to share information about exposure to agents, but it must be done if relapse is to be avoided.

I asked several formerly addicted healthcare professionals who required surgery or anesthesia about the need for full disclosure to their treatment teams prior to receiving potentially addictive medications. Mike, a former dentist who has twenty years of sobriety, was involved in an automobile accident and suffered three broken ribs. "I'm confident about my recovery. I'm not one to avoid my problems; I would rather be confronted with it." Mike told the paramedics who treated him on the scene that he was in recovery and that he wanted to avoid exposure to narcotics if possible. "I tried to avoid triggering agents, but the pain was so severe that I couldn't." For Mike, the exposure didn't trigger a relapse and he was able to avoid exposure on subsequent surgeries through a combination of local anesthesia and non-narcotic analgesics. "They gave me rib blocks with local anesthesia for the thoracotomy and it worked great."

Sarah, a nurse in recovery for less than one year, went to the dentist and was told she required a root canal, the direct result of her addiction to methamphetamines. "I asked that when the procedure was done I not be sent home with a prescription for opiates. I also asked that the midazolam be given before the opiate for induction so that I would not remember the high." Instead of going home after leaving the dentist's office, Sarah went straight to a 12-step meeting. "I told my sponsor what was going on and she was concerned that I might want to get high after getting anesthesia, so she insisted that she pick me up after the procedure. We went for coffee and then to the meeting where I was able to talk about the experience with other people who could relate to what I was going through."

Pam, a radiologist in recovery for three years, was unable to avoid exposure to triggering agents during her surgery. "I had a double mastectomy and lymph node dissection. I was told that I would not be able to go without narcotics, because of the extent of my surgery. I asked for no triggers, but I was told I needed the meds for the initial post-op period. I did not want fentanyl, because I was concerned that I would relapse, but they gave it to me anyway. I also asked for ketorolac (a non-narcotic, non-steroidal anti-inflammatory medication similar to ibuprofen that is given intravenously) post-op instead of hydrocodone, but my surgeon was concerned about bleeding and wouldn't let the anesthesiologist give it to me."

Despite the extensive surgery and postoperative pain, Pam was able to avoid relapse. "I knew as soon as they wrote the prescription for me in the postoperative treatment unit that I was in trouble. I wasn't in pain, but I wanted the medication so badly." Pam went with her husband to fill the prescription and immediately told him to empty the bottle and hide the pills. "I told him that he had to keep track of when I take them, he couldn't let me take them more often than it said on the script and he had to hide the pills. Better yet, he had to keep them with him, because I would go looking for them and I would find them and, if I found them, there was a good chance that I would take them." There were refills authorized on the prescription so Pam asked her husband to give the bottle to her sponsor to hold. "She's been in the group for a lot more time than I have and she can handle it. Even with three years I'm still scared to death of relapse and I don't want that to happen."

Not everyone is so firmly entrenched in recovery as Pam, however. Willie, the nurse educator we discussed, admitted that he has relapsed twice. "Both times were related to injuries. The first time was while I was on the job in an ICU. I was assisting in turning a 600-pound patient and injured my shoulder. When they treated me, I was honest about my disease and that I had successfully taken tramadol for short periods without problems during my recovery." Because he had been honest and up-front with the physician's assistant who treated him, Willie did not receive a prescription for anything that could potentially trigger a relapse. "Unfortunately, I had access and got what I wanted from a friend. Eventually I ended up back at square one and required detoxification and inpatient treatment."

Willie's second relapse was after a fall. "I slipped on some ice and re-injured my shoulder. I had moved since the first relapse, so I had a new doctor and I didn't tell him about my addiction. He gave me hydrocodone and I told myself that it was okay for me to take it because I was in pain. Each time I relapsed I had quit doing the things that I needed to do: I had stopped attending meetings, stopped reading the Big Book. I eventually told my doctor the truth and he helped me get into treatment yet again."

Some healthcare professionals in early recovery may use the need for a potentially painful procedure or surgery as an excuse to relapse. Marvin, an obstetrician, is now seven years out from his initial inpatient treatment. "I relapsed during my first year out. I thank God that I had lost my license, otherwise I would probably be dead."

Marvin's original addiction, he revealed, "started out with butorphanol tartrate, but that didn't really do it for me and it wasn't long before I picked up any narcotic I could find and injected it. Fentanyl was available on the labor floor, so that's what I used most of the time." Marvin obtained most of his fentanyl from the automated machine the anesthesiologists used to store the drugs used to provide labor analgesia. "There was no way I should have been allowed access to that machine. If the pharmacist would have checked the inventory more frequently I would have been caught much sooner."

Marvin was addicted to fentanyl for six months before his partners arranged an intervention that resulted in his admission to an inpatient treatment facility in Pennsylvania. Because of the high volume of narcotics missing from the dispensary, Marvin's case was reported to the State and his license was suspended pending investigation. "By the time the State became involved, I was already in treatment, so they turned my case over to the physician's health program with the understanding that I would have to complete a course of inpatient treatment successfully and be participating in a monitoring program before they would reinstate my license to practice."

It is not uncommon for addicts in early recovery to "hit the wall" at some point during the first year of sobriety and this is when the risk for relapse is highest. "I had completed the three-month inpatient treatment program and I was involved in weekly group therapy with other healthcare professionals who were in similar programs such as I was. I also went to individual therapy once a week." Despite mandated participation in one or more mutual help groups, such as Alcoholics or Narcotics Anonymous, Marvin refused to go. "I was compliant with the program insomuch as I attended the therapy sessions and provided clean urine samples, but I wasn't really in recovery. I was just waiting for an opportunity to use again."

Marvin's opportunity came nine months after his admission to the inpatient treatment facility. "I had these awful pains in my rectum. It's unlikely that this was the result of anal sex, so I had no idea what was going on." Marvin had developed a rectal tear from the constipating effects of chronic narcotic abuse and required surgical correction. "The surgical resident who saw me in the PACU [post-anesthesia care unit, also commonly called the recovery room, where patients are monitored after surgery and before being discharged home] told me he'd never seen such a large tear and gave me a prescription for 100 hydrocodone."

Marvin had no structured plan in place to avoid temptation and relapse. "I held the meds myself. I had already decided that I had had enough of this 'recovery' business and, in retrospect, relapsed long before I actually took the meds." For Marvin, picking up the drugs and choosing to take them was the end result of several months of compliance with a program that did not involve recovery. "Abstinence is not recovery. Don't let anyone tell you that it is," he declared.

With access to large quantities of his drug of choice and a license to use them, Marvin began taking two or three times the prescribed amount in an attempt to get high. "All I got was depressed. The dysphoria caused by the medication bordered on suicidal depression. I never got the high I was looking for and I felt horrible about wasting all that clean time." Marvin was honest with the other members of his group and was able to move forward with their support and encouragement. "One of the guys in my group who lives near me is an alcoholic and he dragged me to a meeting right after the therapy session that day."

From Marvin's example we can see that healthcare professionals in early recovery can make postoperative plans that include preventing relapse as a goal. Equally dangerous is the absence of a plan when faced with the need for exposure to triggering agents. The disease of addiction is a chronic one and the success of any initial treatment is not a cure. Once the disease has been brought under control, much in the same way that a newly diagnosed diabetic may be hospitalized to achieve glycemic control and then discharged on a regimen of medications and further outpatient management, continued treatment is necessary to maintain that control. Healthcare professionals who avoid relapse almost always have specific relapse-prevention plans in place. Despite experiencing cravings and, in some cases, a desire to relapse after exposure, these individuals can successfully avoid relapse through participation in mutual self-help groups such as Alcoholics or Narcotics Anonymous.

When Returning to Work Is Not an Option

Despite the potential for success, not every healthcare professional is given the opportunity to return to clinical practice, even when s/he is seemingly well focused and strong in his or her recovery. Jacob, an anesthesiologist, spent thirty-four months dealing with the consequences of his addiction. He was first caught diverting fentanyl just a few weeks after he finished his residency program. After an intervention and a call to his state's physician health program, Jacob was sent to an inpatient treatment facility that specialized in the treatment of addicted healthcare professionals.

Jacob followed the guidelines and rules they'd set, he told me. He relinquished his license, because his legal counsel told him it was only for a year. However, since he did not have a medical license,

Jacob was told that he would not be able to return to his job after he was discharged from the inpatient training program. He felt they basically fired him and he couldn't even begin to look for another job.

But after twelve months, the medical board had still not scheduled a hearing to review Jacob's request for reinstatement. Jacob's wife didn't make enough to support their family, so the couple began borrowing money to cover necessities and monthly bills as well as the enormous cost of treatment and legal fees. He quickly used up all the credit available on his credit cards.

As months turned into years, Jacob kept going to meetings and relying on the strength of his sober network to keep him focused as he waited for his hearing. Many people, Jacob told me, discussed whether returning to the anesthesia field was the best option for him. But despite that talk, Jacob felt that anesthesiology was the right thing for him to do, a decision supported by his wife and his caseworker at the state physician health program.

Thirty-four months after he voluntarily surrendered his medical license pending review by the state medical board, Jacob was granted the opportunity to present his case. During the hearing, Jacob's lawyer made a compelling case for the reinstatement of Jacob's license, supported by testimony from his caseworker from the physician's health program, his sponsor, several character witnesses and members of his family. Jacob relayed to me that although his wife's testimony evoked emotional reactions from those present, he felt the board members had already made their decision prior to the hearing.

The questions Jacob was asked related to his family history and adolescence. The board wanted to know about Jacob's activities and drug use as a child and teenager. The board also focused on his present condition, stressing the fact that he could have inflicted harm on his patients and not even know it. Jacob felt sure the board would deny his request to reinstate his license and he was surprised when he was told the board's decision was in his favor—but with strict conditions. As he and I discussed the conditions, Jacob relayed to me that he felt he would have been better off with an outright denial of his request.

In this case, the medical board did not want this physician to return to the clinical practice of medicine. The conditions attached to the reinstatement of his medical license included a prohibition against ever practicing anesthesiology, pain management or any medical specialty that required direct handling of or dispensing controlled substances and he was prohibited from obtaining a DEA license. Additionally, the board attached specific work hour restrictions to his license, including restrictions on overnight call, making retraining in another specialty, even in today's climate of resident work hour restrictions, very difficult. The majority of specialty training programs would not allow a trainee to work part time or abstain from on call hours. Jacob expressed that he felt limited to working at walk-in clinics or doing insurance physicals. Additionally, the board increased Jacob's urine monitoring—an added high cost Jacob must pay himself. It seems that even though the medical board reinstated Jacob's license, they placed so many restrictions on it that they have effectively prevented him from practicing medicine.

We must assume that the primary function and goal of the medical board was to protect the public and that it considered Jacob's return to clinical practice to be a threat to public safety. Perhaps they had made up their minds, as Jacob suggested, before the hearing began. Perhaps when they were presented with considerable evidence supporting reinstatement they crafted an alternative judgment that they felt worked for all parties, both protecting the public and allowing Jacob to practice medicine, albeit within the very narrow confines of their ruling.

Changing Careers

Not every healthcare professional who enters treatment for addiction does so with the goal of returning to his chosen field. Some may decide, after becoming sober, that returning to work is not a realistic option if they wish to remain in recovery. The disease of addiction is strong and the risks to both the healthcare professional and his or her patients are high should relapse occur. Sometimes it makes sense to leave the medical field altogether.

Most of the reports and studies which have examined this issue in detail focus on the overwhelmingly positive outcomes that specially designed treatment programs have been able to achieve. A success rate of 72 to 90 percent of healthcare professionals who remain relapse free and working in the healthcare field five years after entering treatment is impressive, but what about the 10 to 28 percent who do not?[6] What happens to the healthcare professional who, despite the existence of a highly structured and effective program, cannot remain sober? What happens to the healthcare professional who is encouraged to retrain in another "less risky" specialty? Are the rates of relapse really less for some specialties? What about the professional who does not have the financial resources to pay for the very expensive inpatient treatment and monitoring programs?

Evaluating the prospects for a safe return to clinical practice by healthcare professionals in recovery can be challenging and sometimes not enough convincing data can be gathered to support such a decision. Rather than make a decision based on incomplete or unconvincing evidence, addictionologists may have to recommend that a healthcare professional consider leaving the field of medicine. One of the stated goals of the medical professionals' alternative-to-discipline programs, in addition to patient safety, is the rehabilitation of addicted healthcare providers. As such, most participants in these programs are eventually given the opportunity to return to clinical practice, as long as they are deemed to be in recovery and agree to abide by the terms set forth in the monitoring contract they have signed.

Sometimes, however, the circumstances surrounding particular individuals' addictions suggest they may be at greater risk for relapse. Perhaps they were abusing one of the major narcotics such as fentanyl and, as well, have strong personal or family histories of mental illness. Perhaps they refuse to admit that they are addicted to these medications in the first place or even that they have done anything wrong by diverting medications intended for their patients. Acknowledgement is the first step in the long process of recovery, but some people are either unable or unwilling to let go. In these cases, the risk for relapse may be too great and if these people are anesthesia care providers or involved in emergency medicine, they may be encouraged to find "less risky" fields in which to retrain.

The Internist Who Used to Be an Anesthesiologist

Lloyd is currently practicing internal medicine as a hospitalist in a small community hospital. Though he began his medical career as an anesthesiologist, he became addicted to fentanyl during the second year of his residency. Lloyd was discovered diverting fentanyl by an attending physician who noticed Lloyd's strange behavior during a case and reported it to the residency program director. "Apparently he thought I was acting strangely. Maybe I was, but it's hard to remember very many details about that time in my life. It wasn't so long ago, but I really want to put it behind me and get on with what I have to do."

Lloyd was treated as an inpatient for ten weeks and then discharged into an intensive inpatient follow-up program. "Even though they had 'suggested' that I should retrain in a different field, I had already completed three years of training and there was no way I wanted to start over. They called my program director and all of a sudden the residency program had this 'one strike, you're out' policy. I couldn't believe it. It was like, 'Thanks so much for your work over the last few years. Here's the door; don't let it hit you in the ass on your way out.'" He was encouraged to retrain in a different specialty. "This was not my choice and, to be quite frank, I'm not happy about it at all." Even three years later, Lloyd remains bitter about the way he was treated by both the physician health program and his former residency program director. "After that I really didn't have a choice. I had completed an intern year in medicine, so I figured it would be easiest to go back into medicine and finish the last two years of the residency."

Lloyd graduated from his new residency program in medicine and was able to obtain a position as a hospitalist. "I know, I know. I really should be grateful that I'm alive and that no one got hurt because of me and that I still have my medical license, but it's hard when you really don't like what you do every day. I feel like I was forced into this." Lloyd is still monitored by the physician health program he signed on with during his ten-week stay at the inpatient treatment center and he is required to attend weekly meetings with his group therapist as well as submit specimens for urine testing on a regular basis. His story is unique in that he was not allowed the opportunity to attempt to return to clinical anesthesia before being asked to retrain in a different specialty. Though this is not unprecedented, most professionals who are not allowed to return to clinical anesthesia have previously been given that chance and have relapsed.

When these healthcare professionals, physicians, nurses or other healthcare workers are asked to leave their avocations and work in other related but distinctly different fields, this decision should not be made lightly. Often the professional is encouraged to enter a "less risky" specialty, though it is not clear just how much safer alternative fields are. Some have pointed out, and rightly so, that the considerable experience the field of anesthesia has concerning issues related to addiction identification and treatment actually make this a safer environment in which to attempt reentry. Healthcare professionals in recovery who return to the clinical practice of anesthesia in closely monitored settings with full disclosure are more likely to be watched not only by those assigned to monitor their behavior and actions but also by their colleagues. While the statistics suggest that healthcare professionals in some specialties have lower rates of addiction to prescription medications, one cannot assume that someone with a history of addiction will suddenly become less likely to relapse because he or she is practicing in a different field. Forcing someone who has demonstrated that he or she has an increased risk for further substance abuse to retrain in a specialty where his or her colleagues might not understand as much about the natural course of the disease may not be the right choice.

An Addict Who Couldn't Stay Clean

Despite the increased vigilance with which a healthcare professional who returns to clinical practice is monitored, sometimes that is not enough, and this may become clear after just one relapse. Noah was an anesthesia resident in his last weeks of training when he was identified as possibly having a drug problem and sent for an inpatient evaluation. "I got a little too drunk at a pre-graduation party and I guess people noticed. The next week I misplaced some fentanyl and all of a sudden I'm sitting in my program director's office trying to explain to him that I'm not an addict."

Because the volume of fentanyl that Noah had lost was so great, the hospital pharmacy had to report it to the DEA and the state medical board began an investigation. "I spoke to someone at [the state PHP] and they suggested that it would look better for me to get evaluated and have some clean urine to use for my defense. They said it would only be for three days and that it wouldn't prevent me from starting my new job on time." Noah had secured a lucrative partnership track position at a private practice group in the area, but he never got to work a single day there. "I've been drinking and doing cocaine my whole adult life. I guess I didn't realize how long that stuff stays in your system." Noah's first urine screening came up negative for fentanyl metabolites but positive for cocaine. "I spent twelve weeks trying to convince them that I really did lose the fentanyl and that I hadn't injected it or put it away for a rainy day or something like that."

In September, three months after the rest of his classmates had graduated and were well into their first years working as fellows in academic programs or attending anesthesiologists in private practice, Noah returned to his residency program but not to work as a resident. "[The treatment program] must have given me a bad evaluation or something because my case worker at [the physician health program] wasn't too keen on my going back to work." Because there was an investigation being conducted by the state medical board, Noah hired a lawyer who specialized in these types of cases. "I was amazed to find out that there was enough work in this city for two or three of these guys to practice full time just defending doctors in my position. He told me that, because the DEA was involved, it would be a while before they allowed me to return to clinical work and when they said it was okay, then I would have to apply to the anesthesia board for reinstatement as a resident and redo my last clinical year." Noah was hired as a teaching assistant at the residency program he had almost graduated from and waited for the medical board to complete its investigation.

Eighteen months after the investigation began, Noah received notice from the state medical board that he would be allowed to continue his training in clinical anesthesia. He still maintained that he had never used fentanyl and, since he had been compliant with the terms of his monitoring contract with the physician health program, he was given credit for two years of training and was allowed to return to residency to repeat his last year of training.

Since he did not have a medical license and had been practicing as a resident on a limited permit, the state board stipulated that he would apply for and receive a state medical license which would then be revoked based on Noah's admission to "committing professional misconduct as defined by being a habitual user of alcohol or being dependent on or being a habitual user of narcotics, barbiturates, amphetamines, hallucinogens or other drugs having a similar effect or having a psychiatric condition which impairs the licensee's ability to practice medicine." The revocation would be stayed and his license would be put on probation for a period of five years with stipulations that included an aftercare treatment plan, periodic evaluation by a psychiatrist, monitoring by a healthcare professional, random drug testing and supervision at work by a licensed physician. Noah signed an agreement to abide by the stipulations as a condition of obtaining a license to practice medicine and he was allowed to return to clinical practice.

Two months later Noah violated the terms of his probation by "inappropriately obtaining and injecting himself with fentanyl" and was dismissed from his residency program. Despite having spent twenty-three months in a program designed to help him stay sober, Noah was unable to resist the temptation to continue to use drugs. "I can't explain away my actions; I guess they were right to be concerned about me." As outlined in the contract he had signed with the state board of medicine, his license was revoked, making it impossible for him to practice medicine. "My lawyer said that if I wanted to try again I should stay in the program and reapply to the board after I have a few more years of sobriety under my belt, but I just don't have it in me anymore."

Noah has spent the last three years working in a field unrelated to medicine. "I still have my degree; they can't take that away from me. Since I no longer have a medical license I can't practice medicine, but there are plenty of jobs available for people with the intimate knowledge I have of how the system works. With the changes that are happening in healthcare, more and more people with MDs are leaving clinical practice anyway, so I don't usually have to explain why I don't practice clinically."

The system is not perfect, but in Noah's case it worked to protect both the physician and the public without depriving either of the opportunity for a second chance. Despite the absence of any evidence to suggest that he was actively using during the prolonged investigation by the state medical board, the physician health program that was monitoring him chose to keep him out of clinical practice rather than allow him to go back to work. Perhaps his case worker had a hunch that something was not quite right.

It is alarming that our ability to monitor healthcare professionals in recovery is as imperfect as it is, but eventually the decision has to be made one way or another. In Noah's case, the doubts held by the physician health program caseworker coupled with the probationary status of his medical license resulted in his removal from the practice of medicine when his relapse was detected. Had the circumstances of his recovery been different, it is possible that he might have been given a third chance, but it seems he is not willing to maintain his sobriety in order to achieve this goal. When we spoke I asked Noah if he was still using. "I still drink, maybe less than I did when I was younger, but I don't see any problem with it. Every once in a while I'll do some blow, but that's it. I'd rather live like this and not be a doctor than have to put up with all the monitoring and therapy crap that I'd have to do to keep my license."

After Twenty-Five Years Under the Influence

Forgiving and offering second chances are commendable. To believe that someone who has stumbled will be able to pick him or herself up and move forward shows compassion. We hope that these people will not stumble again, but sometimes to avoid this, it requires a change of direction. The successes of the healthcare professionals' treatment programs are impressive, but somehow lost in the numbers are the stories of the people who have survived their addictions because they have been prevented from returning to the fields of medicine or nursing. The minority of cases involving individuals who have not been able to return to clinical practice should not be seen as a failure of the treatment programs. The only true failures of the system are the individuals who die or injure patients before they can be identified or relapses that result in harm to providers or their patients. Former healthcare professionals in recovery and in new fields are alive and unable to harm patients.

Bruce began his career in emergency medicine under the influence of alcohol, marijuana and cocaine. "I had used drugs and alcohol since high school, smoked pot pretty much every day in medical school, used cocaine regularly as a resident and drank heavily when I wasn't at work." Because he had always been abusing, there were no changes in behavior to notice. Perhaps because he was reasonably competent or perhaps because nobody wanted to say anything, nobody complained about his work either. "I showed up on time, did what I needed to do and then left to get high or drunk. For me, emergency medicine was the ultimate job. I loved what I did and I was very good at it. Best of all, I didn't have to take it home with me. When I walked out that door at the end of the shift my time belonged to nobody but me until it was time to come back."

Bruce was reported to the state medical board after he was arrested attempting to purchase cocaine from an undercover police officer. After his release from jail, Bruce was allowed to enter an alternative-to-discipline program and spent three months at an inpatient rehabilitation program. "After I detoxed, I realized that it had been twenty-five years since I had been sober. Can you imagine that? I had experienced the past two and a half decades under the influence."

While he was an inpatient, Bruce received notification from the state board that his license would be suspended pending a hearing on his recovery status. The physician health program in which he was participating suggested that, given his extensive drug history, he should take some time away from practice before applying to have his license reinstated. "Even though I wasn't busted at work, they were concerned that my extracurricular activities would interfere with my ability to practice competently. They said that nobody would believe that anyone could turn around a twenty-five-year drug habit in three months."

Faced with free time, Bruce decided to go back to school. "I applied to law school and by the time I heard from the state medical board that they were ready to hear my case, I was already enrolled." Bruce opted to finish his law degree rather than attempt a return to medicine. "I realized that everything I loved about emergency medicine was perfect for me when I was high but being sober it didn't seem so attractive. The work is hard and the hours are long and I suspected that if I had gone back I probably would have been using within a month anyway." For Bruce, the perspective he was able to appreciate after being sober for an extended period of time made his choice to leave the practice of medicine an easy one. He now works as a lawyer representing physicians who have had their licenses suspended or revoked for diversion.

In many cases, the ultimate decision regarding the return to clinical practice does not depend on the sobriety of the individual healthcare professional but on other factors. The risk of death when relapse occurs in formerly addicted healthcare professionals is high, as is the risk for injury to the patients for whom they care. The decision to allow these individuals to return to clinical practice should be made only when all of the factors that can contribute to relapse have been evaluated by qualified personnel.

PART V

WHAT NEEDS TO BE DONE

Chapter 13

Proactive Measures to Prevent Harm

The use of recreational pharmaceuticals can affect job performance, even if the employee is not acutely intoxicated. Deficits in reaction time and the ability to concentrate on repetitive tasks may persist long after the acute effects of intoxication have worn off. This is especially concerning for employees who must perform at very high levels on a regular basis, such as those in the healthcare industry. Many employers who operate in safety-sensitive industries, such as aviation, railroad transportation and even retail warehouse stores, have chosen to institute "drug-free workplace" policies designed to reduce the risk for errors and harm related to impaired performance. Despite a proven record of decreased incidents related to impairment after the institution of such policies, for some reason workplace drug screening for all medical personnel remains a contentious issue.

Fabricating Drug Test Results

It is a bright late summer afternoon toward the end of August. The streets of this town in New Jersey are deserted, as most have abandoned the oppressive heat for the cooling breezes of the shore, and I find a parking spot easily. Those who have remained behind apparently prefer to stay indoors and there is nobody to watch as I quickly move from the comfort of my air-conditioned car through the thick humid air and into the dim light of the establishment I have come to visit.

The door closes with a loud click behind me and it takes a moment for my eyes to adjust from the bright sunlight. Jimmy is leaning against the wall behind a counter, watching a game show on the television mounted to the wall behind me. I introduce myself and explain why I'm there and a wide grin appears on his face. "These days you have to be an idiot to fail a pre-employment screening," he says. "We have anything you need to pass any test and I can tell you which kit you need, depending on what you've been taking." Jimmy pulls out a number of different bags of what appear to be herbs or tea leaves. "If you're into pills and you want to keep getting high while you're looking for a new job, just make a pot of this and drink it over four hours before your test. You'll pass even if you're high while you're peeing."

Apparently the best-selling variety is the one for marijuana. "I get a lot of potheads who are heavy into it and have a short time to get ready for the test." He pushes what looks like marijuana in a plastic baggie across the glass counter. "This stuff won't get you high, but it will keep the man from knowing what you're doing when you're not on the job, if you know what I mean. It's also good for tobacco too. Every once in a while I get some suit in here who smokes that brown shit and wants to drop a clean urine for an insurance physical. I get all kinds in here, man."

Pre-Employment Drug Screenings

It is better to avoid hiring an individual who is using drugs in the first place, but drug tests are necessary. When passing a drug test is a condition for employment with a particular hospital or practice, a healthcare professional who is actively using drugs has ample time to prepare. For many highly motivated individuals, simply not taking the drug for a period of time will produce a negative result. For those who are unable or unwilling to stop using, an Internet search provides multiple methods for circumventing the process. A motivated individual can find "clean" urine for sale and even artificial genitalia of the appropriate skin color for exams that must be witnessed. To get around this issue, some hospitals offer prospective new employees positions which include probationary periods during which they are randomly tested for drugs of abuse. While some residency training programs and hospitals do require pre-employment drug screenings, very few training programs or non-military hospitals continue to test employees after they have been hired.

For-Cause Drug Screenings

Some hospital policies include drug screenings which are conducted only when probable cause or reasonable suspicion of drug use exists. The triggers for these types of tests are different across institutions, as there are no national standards, and may range from suspicious behavior to a "near-miss" or actual patient harm. If a physician, nurse or any healthcare professional is thought to be behaving in a manner which suggests that he or she may be impaired and a drug screening is administered, the suspected professional is usually removed from clinical work until the results of the test return.

When suspicious behavior triggers the inquiry, especially if it is the behavior of a physician or someone in a managerial or executive position, an investigation is conducted to obtain corroborating evidence prior to confronting the individual to request a urine or hair sample. Drug screenings, which are administered after a defined incident such as a medication administration error, loss of controlled substances or patient harm, usually do not require such an investigation before collecting a sample for analysis.

Drug screenings have limitations in the post-incident setting. While a positive result indicates that the individual has used drugs at some point in the past, it does not necessarily imply intoxication at work or even that the incident which triggered the drug screening resulted from impairment. If the hospital has a drug-free workplace policy, then a positive result on a post-incident screening would trigger a defined response, likely resulting in an intervention and the referral of the healthcare professional to an impatient facility for evaluation.

Ariel, a scrub technician, works at a hospital with just such a policy. "Not too long ago we had one of our anesthesiologists lose a bag of controlled drugs (which at Ariel's institution are commonly carried in a locked satchel by the anesthesiologist or CRNA responsible for them) and we all had to pee in a cup." The anesthesiologist and the CRNA Ariel was working with, as well as anyone who could have possibly had access to the drugs, were tested to rule out addiction as the motivation for the theft. The fact that the drugs could have been stolen for another reason is not lost on Ariel. "Around here there's a lot of money in these drugs. You can walk out the front door and sell them to the first person you see without any problem. Probably make a lot of money too."

Regardless of the reason for the theft, the CRNA involved with the case ended up becoming a casualty of the investigation. "The way I hear it, she was smoking pot and it came up in her urine. Now, I know that's not what they were looking for, but that's what they found and they had to do something about it, didn't they?" The CRNA, though not impaired and not implicated in the theft of the drugs, was removed from her clinical duties and sent for an evaluation at an inpatient facility. "They fired her after that; no chance she'll ever come back to work here anymore. Now if it was the anesthesiologist physician things would be different, I tell you. Docs get special treatment when it comes to things like that." Ironically, the anesthesiologist involved was also let go from her clinical position and no longer works for the hospital, though apparently for different reasons.

Random Drug Screenings

Random drug testing works best to increase workplace safety by reducing the number of accidents related to on-the-job drug or alcohol use. When coupled with a strict policy of zero tolerance for drug or alcohol use, the addition of random urine testing to the workplace can have a positive deterrent effect as well. This has been shown to be true in every branch of the United States military as well as most constituents of the Department of Transportation (DOT), the Federal Transit Administration (FTA), the Federal Aviation Administration (FAA) and the Federal Railroad Administration (FRA). The FTA reported rate of transit fatalities from all causes was 12.4 per 100 million vehicle miles in 1994. The next year, the year they implemented a policy of random drug testing among federal transit workers, the rate dropped to 8.0 deaths per 100 million vehicle miles. By 2003 that number was down to 5.7 deaths per 100 million vehicle miles.[1]

Almost immediately after the implementation of such a policy in these federally managed programs, a statistically significant decline in the number of deaths was evident. Given the parallels between healthcare professionals and the employees in these safety-sensitive industries, where a single person's job performance can have a significant impact on a large number of people, it would seem prudent to implement a program of random testing of all healthcare professionals. Such a policy would no doubt have the dual effect of both reducing the incidences of the diversion of controlled substances and detecting an individual early in the course of addiction, before harming the person or someone else.

I spoke with Edward, the medical review officer for a large group anesthesia practice, who related, "We have contracts at quite a number of facilities and not all of them have the same philosophy when it comes to on-the-job drug testing. Some of the state-run facilities use random testing. It's a difficult argument, because some of these drugs can be in your system long after you're no longer impaired. For people who use it on a regular basis, marijuana can stay in your system for up to thirty days; does that mean you're impaired thirty days after you last smoked?"

Urine testing is still the cornerstone for monitoring and documenting abstinence in the recovering healthcare professional, but how does it work as a therapeutic tool? Edward conveyed, "Random urine tests are a very strong tool. They help motivate the healthcare professional in recovery to maintain sobriety as well as to provide accountability. They also probably serve as a deterrent. I'm sure there are a few people who never try to divert these medications in the first place, because they know there's a pretty good chance they're going to get caught."

If a policy of random drug testing is to be imposed, it must be implemented in accordance with Substance Abuse Mental Health Services Administration (SAMHSA) guidelines and the protocol for proper chain of custody should be strictly followed. This means that micturition must be witnessed. Someone must actually watch the employee provide the specimen for analysis. Once it is collected, each specimen should be split into two samples, with half of the urine tested and half frozen for subsequent testing if indicated.

Drug testing is then conducted via radioimmunoassay (RIA), which is sensitive but not specific, meaning it is used to rule *out* drug use. A negative result on the rather sensitive RIA test is taken to mean that the person is not using any of the drugs that were tested for. A positive result *may* indicate that the person has been using drugs, but the RAI test is not specific so drug use must then be confirmed using the gas chromatography/mass spectrometry (GC/MS) technique. This is why the original specimen is split—half is saved in the event of a positive result that needs confirmation. This second test is used to rule *in* drug use. When testing healthcare professionals with access to unique medications, it is important to remember that many of these drugs are not included in a routine urine toxicology screening. For instance, specific requests must be made to include drugs such as a fentanyl or propofol.

For this strategy to be an effective deterrent to workplace drug use, healthcare professionals must first be aware of the policy and understand that the testing will be unannounced and completely random. Each employee should have an equal chance of being selected to provide a sample, regardless of the last time a person was tested. It is important that the screenings occur on a truly random basis, as any predictability will reduce the deterrent effect. It is also important that employees not get the impression that they will not be tested for a period of time after a sample is taken, as some may take this opportunity to use drugs, thinking that they will not be tested in the post-screening period. Typically each employee is assigned a number which is randomly selected by a computer at regular intervals. It is also possible to collect a specimen from everybody in the department and then randomly select which samples are tested.

Testing Recovering Addicts

Urine and hair testing are still the cornerstones for monitoring and documenting abstinence in recovering addicts. In the case of a formerly addicted healthcare professional who is in recovery, urine or hair testing should be performed more frequently. The value of random testing as a therapeutic tool in this population is clear: It has a significant deterring effect on drug use and can identify a relapse earlier than relying on workplace deterioration. Specific requests must be made to include drugs such as fentanyl that a recovering healthcare professional may have access to or has a history of abusing, as the routine drug screenings typically do not include these drugs. If the individual is a reentrant on naltrexone, the drug screening needs to include an assay for naltrexone as well. If there is reason to suspect that the individual may be abusing propofol, a specific request must be made to test for propofol-specific metabolites.

In order to use these tools to detect drug abuse, you need to know the suspected drug's half-life, the extent to which it is modified by metabolism in the body and how it is eliminated. For a drug like fentanyl, the primary route of elimination is metabolic. Norfentanyl, a fentanyl metabolite, can be detected in the urine up to ninety-six hours after small (100 microgram) doses of fentanyl. The primary metabolites of morphine (Morphine-3-glucuronide) and of meperidine (normeperidine) can be detected in urine for up to seventy-two hours after administration. A regular fentanyl user should have detectable fentanyl in the urine for three to five days after the last time the user ingested the drug, though there are some "recovering" addicts who reported that regular fentanyl abuse was not detected on routine urine tests.

Kenneth, a nurse in treatment for fentanyl abuse, reported just such a phenomenon. "I was treated for addiction to oxycodone several years ago and had nine years of clean time before I relapsed." When Kenneth started using narcotics again, he stayed away from the pills he had preferred in the past and instead began using fentanyl. "I got a job in the intensive care unit and we had access to a lot of fentanyl. I wasn't used to working in such an intense setting and I started using the fentanyl on a regular basis to settle my nerves."

Shortly after he started diverting fentanyl, a pharmacist noticed a discrepancy in the stock and everyone in the unit who had access was tested. "They made us all pee in a cup but nobody came up positive. I figured I was in the clear so I continued to use." It wasn't long before another discrepancy was noticed, but this time Kenneth was asked to provide a hair sample for analysis, which came back positive.

Because the half-lives of most of the agents typically abused by healthcare professionals are so short, hair testing, which is more sensitive, should be included with urine testing. The analysis of hair samples obtained from an individual under the same chain-of-custody guidelines as for urine or blood samples can detect chronic use over a longer period of time. Depending on the length of the hair, it is possible to test exposure over a period of time measured in months rather than hours or days. Hair can serve as a marker of chronic exposure because of the way drugs of abuse or their metabolites are incorporated into the structure of the hair follicle over time as the hair grows. While it is unclear how this actually happens, it is likely that the drugs or their metabolites passively diffuse from blood capillaries into the hair cells as the hair grows. Alternatively, these chemicals may be deposited onto the hair after it has been formed through contact with sweat or other secretions.

The techniques used today to detect the presence of drugs of abuse are so sensitive that extremely small levels of the drugs can be detected. Even though minute quantities of substances in the hair of individuals suspected of illicit drug use can be used as evidence to confirm suspected relapse, there are certain limitations to the use of this technique. One is the need for hair to test. An individual who presents for a hair test after having trimmed or shaved his or her hair entirely should be considered suspect for drug abuse, but hair can be obtained from alternative areas such as the underarms, pubic area, chest or thigh. Just as with urine tests, the possibility for contamination exists and it is possible to produce positive test results after environmental exposure to particular drugs. Because of this, the individual taking the sample should thoroughly wash his or her hands and wear gloves when obtaining the sample.

Naltrexone, Buprenorphine and Other Tools

Naltrexone is a drug which fully antagonizes the effects of narcotic drugs with abuse potential such as hydrocodone and fentanyl. By preventing a person from experiencing a high should he or she self-administer narcotics, naltrexone has the potential to prevent return to chronic use should an addict relapse, as well as to protect against a fatal overdose. Another drug, naloxone, also has been shown to reduce cravings in alcoholics and recovering healthcare professionals who wish to return to clinical practice are often required to use it. Taking naltrexone is not sobriety, but it does offer a significant safety net for recovering healthcare providers much in the same way that the monitoring programs promote abstinence until motivation for recovery becomes internal. Because of this, its use should be considered part of a comprehensive program of recovery.

Naltrexone can be administered daily via the oral route, once a month in the form of an intramuscular depot injection or through an extended release naltrexone pellet that can be implanted subcutaneously and provide continuous clinically effective levels of naltrexone for three to four months.

In some cases, healthcare professionals may be treated with narcotic medications such as methadone. First synthesized during World War II because of a shortage of morphine and introduced in 1947 as an analgesic, methadone is currently used for the treatment of narcotic addiction or chronic pain management. Since its effects last up to twenty-four hours, high doses of methadone can be used to block the effects of other narcotics and prevent the symptoms of withdrawal. Since tolerance and dependence to methadone can result, abrupt cessation of methadone maintenance can precipitate a withdrawal syndrome. Methadone administration discourages the use of other narcotics, but maintenance therapy is associated with neurocognitive deficits and may not be appropriate for all healthcare professionals, especially those in specialties such as anesthesiology where reduced vigilance would not be acceptable.

There is a considerable difference between the level of vigilance expected of the anesthesia care provider and the podiatrist, so recovery based in narcotic replacement may be acceptable for some healthcare professionals. Recovery while maintained on methadone is not considered abstinence-based recovery and is not allowed by many monitoring programs.

Initially marketed in the United States as an analgesic, the semi-synthetic narcotic buprenorphine was approved for the treatment of narcotic addiction in 2002. Buprenorphine has a long duration of action, much like methadone, and can be administered orally, but it is associated with much less respiratory depression and is considered to have an improved safety profile with less risk of fatal overdose. Because of these qualities, healthcare professionals in recovery who are unable to remain sober without the assistance of narcotic replacement therapy are more likely to be maintained on buprenorphine.

Educating Healthcare Professionals

Prevention is the most desirable method of approaching the problem of drug abuse in our society's healthcare professionals. Educating the community regarding the potential for substance abuse among healthcare providers plays an important role in this process. The hope is that widespread education regarding the extremely dangerous nature of these medications and the risk of addiction may serve as both a deterrent and an aid in the early detection of afflicted individuals. Unfortunately, little if any attention is paid to this topic in the curriculums of the nation's medical schools and training programs.

The age at which new healthcare professionals begin their schooling and early training and the culture of acceptance toward drugs to which they have likely been exposed puts these individuals at high risk for the development of addiction before they even begin independent practice. In fact, most impaired professionals report addictive behavior that existed while they were medical or nursing students, if not before.

I believe the lack of a standardized curriculum on this topic is appalling. Any student who wishes to attend medical, dental or optometry school must take certain pre-medical courses and pass a nationally standardized entrance exam: the MCAT (Medical College Admissions Test) for medical schools, the DAT (Dental Admissions Test) for dental schools and the OAT (Optometry Admissions Test) for optometry schools. These standardized entrance requirements are irrespective of what state an applicant is applying from or where a school is based and serve the purpose of culling the herd of applicants so that only the most qualified are admitted into the various programs. Once these students begin their training, the standard curriculum continues and students are expected to pass a series of standardized licensing exams. So why is there such a variance when it comes to the structure of education in addiction medicine?

As a medical student I received no formal training in the treatment of addiction among my patients and no lectures on physician impairment. It appears that this has not changed significantly in the past ten years. The first step in educating the healthcare professionals' community should come during the training process. Without a firm basis of understanding these issues, subsequent education in the form of brief lectures or yearly seminars carries less influence. The goal should be for every healthcare professional to graduate from a school or training program with a firm and realistic understanding of the potential for addiction in colleagues and the ability to recognize this impairment when it occurs.

While as a group the medical community has done a dismal job so far of educating its members on addiction, there are some specialty groups that recognize the long and pervasive history of addiction in medical personnel and have put in place educational programs specific to the experience of their members. The American Association of Nurse Anesthetists (AANA) became the first organization to address these issues formally through both the creation of an educational program designed to reduce the impact of addiction on their specialty and a policy shift away from punishment of addicted nurses and toward treatment. Diana Quinlan, a certified registered nurse anesthetist (CRNA), supervised the creation of educational programs designed to provide a safety net for CRNAs who had become addicted to anesthetic agents.

Responding to the same issues among the physician members of its ranks, the American Society of Anesthesiologists (ASA) organized a Task Force on Chemical Dependence led by Bill Arnold which attempted to provide practical answers to the problem of drug addiction in anesthesia personnel.[2] The specialty of anesthesia can be considered the first both to acknowledge that this issue exists and to work toward finding a solution to the problem. Bill Arnold and Diana Quinlan, through their work within the ASA and AANA, began the campaign to educate anesthesia care providers about the dangers of substance abuse.

Since this campaign began, a number of media, film and video programs have been designed to bring the issue of addiction in medical practice to the forefront. The most popular and well-known among them is the *Wearing Masks* series of seven films warning of the potential for substance abuse in anesthesia providers. This series of educational films is now funded entirely by the AANA in response to the death of Jan Stewart, former president of the AANA, who died of an overdose in 2002. The *Wearing Masks* series is distributed by All Anesthesia: The Coalition for the Prevention of Addiction in Anesthesia and is available free of charge. Sarah Stewart Gomes, the daughter of Jan Stewart, created *About Wellness*, a powerful video message that warns viewers of the toll that addiction can take on nurse anesthetists and their loved ones. This video is frequently used by those charged with creating awareness of addiction and other obstacles to wellness among the members of their practice group. Formal educational programs such as this are used by medical departments, physician groups and hospital administrators to ensure awareness of the issue of workplace drug addiction among healthcare professionals.

There are a number of other educational videos that directly address the issue of substance abuse in medical personnel and many are used as part of programs of education for individuals in training or newly hired personnel. Some programs have specifically organized sessions for the spouses or partners of the trainees to view one or more of these films together so that they will be more likely to learn the signs of addiction in their companions.

Despite the increased number of hours that have been devoted to the education of healthcare professionals, the rate of substance abuse in this population appears to be growing. I strongly believe that proactive measures such as random drug testing for all healthcare professionals should be implemented at all levels. The public needs to become involved. Continuing to study and discuss this issue will eventually remove the stigma attached to impairment through addiction, encouraging more addicted healthcare professionals to seek assistance earlier in the course of the disease and empowering those who come in contact with them to speak up sooner.

CONCLUSION

The Need for National Standards and Consistent Policy

I believe that the public has a right to know what they are getting into when they walk through the doors of a hospital or doctor's office. As medical providers move away from the paternalistic attitudes of last century's culture of medicine and expect patients to come to them with more knowledge of their conditions, ready to be active partners in the fights against their diseases, it is appropriate to pull back the curtain from some of medicine's old practices. The unwillingness to address the taboo topic of addiction in the members of society tasked with treating it helped to perpetuate the idea that healthcare professionals are somehow different from everyone else. While the problems that today's healthcare professionals face and the expectations that society makes on them may be unique, the people who choose to train in and ultimately work in these professions do so with the same predisposition to addiction and other diseases as those who don't. To pretend that healthcare providers are somehow immune to addiction is to deny that medical professionals are just as human as the patients for whom they care.

The treatments available to impaired healthcare professionals, especially the programs available to addicted physicians, work. Since we normally do not discuss addiction in this context, the majority of people who are not directly involved have no idea what this treatment involves and are unable to make an informed decision when they are faced with the need to obtain treatment for themselves or a loved one.

Addiction is a chronic, relapsing disease that is often very difficult to treat. It is not something that can be cured, and sending an impaired individual to a traditional twenty-eight-day inpatient program followed by discharge back to the same situation from whence s/he came, with little or no aftercare, does a disservice to the addict as well as to society. Often the costs of such a meager program cannot be covered by addicts in treatment and they are discharged prematurely, only to chronically relapse and require further treatment. Who ultimately pays the price for these failed treatments? Who pays directly for the costs associated with repeated relapse? Who pays the opportunity costs associated with the loss of a productive member of society? What about the costs of caring for this individual when he or she is not in treatment and unable to care for him or herself? What about the costs of treating the injuries, either self-inflicted or inflicted on others by the impaired individual? What about the cost of crime associated with addiction?

Society does not place the same value on the treatment of addictive disorders that it does on the treatment of other serious medical conditions such as diabetes, cancer and heart disease. The very best insurance programs frequently cover only half of the costs of the initial addiction treatment and place unrealistic limits on the amount of aftercare available to patients. This is shortsighted and wrong. If we expect the addict to recover then we have to treat the disease properly and this takes both time and money.

I strongly believe the physician health programs described in this book hold the greatest likelihood of success for any addicted individual, regardless of occupation. It is a long and arduous road to recovery that many are unwilling or unable to take without significant support. It is expensive and inconvenient and, in today's climate of immediate gratification, the period of time required for proper treatment can seem like a lifetime. Unfortunately for the addict who receives inadequate treatment, the price can actually be a lifetime.

What's Wrong with Today's System

There are a number of problems with the healthcare professionals' programs, which I have also attempted to point out, but I believe that these stem not from an underlying inadequacy inherent in the treatment model but rather from poor implementation at various levels along the way of what is, in theory, a great idea. There is a lack of standardized education on identifying impaired healthcare professionals at every level of training. Most medical students receive inadequate education covering how to treat addicted patients and often no discussions at all on the topic of impaired healthcare professionals. This silence adds to the stigma of addiction and hinders early identification and treatment. Since most impairment begins during school or early training and is, in retrospect, evident at that point, changes that reflect this reality need to be made in the curricula of medical, nursing, pharmacy and dental schools as well as in training programs for the allied health professions.

There is no standardized approach to treatment and post-treatment protocols for addicted healthcare professionals among the states and this is a problem. While some states have put in place exemplary programs for the treatment and post-treatment monitoring of impaired healthcare professionals, the standards and practices in other states are lax and inadequate. It is time to move toward a national standard of treatment and monitoring which combines the best parts of programs from states with proven records of success and eliminates the parts that either don't work or are counterproductive.

As we have seen, there is a wide range of policies among the different states regarding certain aspects of treatment of addicted healthcare professionals and this is no longer acceptable. Additionally, there is a wide range of success when it comes to these programs' abilities to rehabilitate addicted healthcare professionals and return them to clinical practice. Some states have been very successful and report that upwards of 90 percent of their program graduates remain relapse free and practicing clinically five years after initial treatment.[1] Other states have closed their programs altogether, claiming that they are ineffective and do little to protect the public. These programs grew out of a desire for the physician and nursing societies to be able to police themselves and protect their members, offering treatment instead of punishment. Since this punishment frequently came in the form of sanctions handed down by the state medical or nursing board, it makes sense that each state would develop its own unique program to deal with the issues that pertain to the health-care professionals in that region. What is necessary now, however, is the creation of a national standard with treatment and monitoring requirements that have been proven to work and that must be observed by all states.

Adopting National Standards

Establishing national standards for treatment and monitoring will ensure that any impaired healthcare professional will be referred to a program that has a proven record of successfully rehabilitating addicts as well as protecting the public. There are currently a number of programs that claim to specialize in the treatment of addicted healthcare professionals, but most do not have enough support for a program solely for healthcare providers. These professional programs often also include police officers, firefighters and, increasingly, pilots as well as members of the general population.

Current models of successful treatment suggest that programs with only healthcare professionals are most effective for this population. Under the current system, addicted healthcare professionals are referred to inpatient programs for their initial treatments based on the experience and connections of their counselors at the impaired professionals' program. Under a more cohesive system based on national standards, addicted healthcare professionals would be referred directly to a national center of excellence with the experience, funding and staffing to provide effective treatment in the proper environment for this population.

After successfully completing the initial inpatient program, an addicted healthcare professional typically returns to his or her home location and is enrolled in a monitoring program with varying requirements and varying lengths. Some states require urine testing and do not recognize the value of hair testing while others combine both random urine and regular hair testing. Some states use a system where the healthcare professional must either dial in to a computer via telephone or use the Internet to find out if he or she is required to submit a specimen for analysis, while others rely on a network of paid urine collectors to contact the participating professionals randomly and request samples. Still other states allow any physician to serve as the urine monitor for an impaired healthcare professional, a practice which can result in less than random sampling, especially if the monitor and the addict have a familiar relationship, as is usually the case. The length of the required monitoring contracts is also not standardized.

Future Directions

It is important to recognize the necessity to develop an impaired healthcare professionals policy that protects all involved parties. An addicted healthcare professional presents a clear and present danger to society through possible negligent practice and diversion of controlled medications. In today's team approach to the delivery of healthcare, any member of the team has the potential to harm patients, not just the physician who may make an incorrect diagnosis, the surgeon who may injure a patient while performing surgery or the anesthesiologist who may harm a patient while under the influence. No longer is it only the nurse who delivers the wrong medication, because she is preoccupied with where she will get her next fix. Now it is also the respiratory technician who does not respond to an airway emergency in a timely manner, because he is under the influence, the pharmacist who dispenses diluted or substituted medication to avoid being caught diverting these medications for personal use and even the patient transporter who inadvertently takes a patient to the wrong location, prolonging treatment or diagnosis, who have the potential to harm. The sick and injured who rely on the knowledge and skill that healthcare professionals possess represent some of the most vulnerable members of society and those who will benefit most from a comprehensive policy.

Under the current structure, impaired professionals are offered the enticement of anonymity coupled with the threat of reporting to the state licensing board as the incentive to seek treatment voluntarily. In reality, enrollment in these programs is hardly voluntary, as non-compliance almost always results in the case being turned over to the state licensing board, the end result of which is usually revocation of the license in question. If an impaired professional wants to retain his or her livelihood and ability to practice, non-compliance is not a realistic option. As a result, there is a strong incentive for impaired professionals to remain compliant with the terms of the treatment program and monitoring contract.

The individuals who successfully complete alternative-to-discipline programs may never come into contact with the licensing board and, as such, may never have such treatment mentioned in their records. A formerly impaired healthcare professional may return to clinical practice without his or her employer or colleagues knowing his or her history of addiction. Proponents of the current structure argue that it is this promise of anonymity that ensures compliance with these programs and therefore increases patient safety. They point out that addiction is a disease of despair and depression; to remove anonymity from the treatment program is tantamount to removing hope of eventual return to "normal" clinical practice and this would doom these programs to failure.

I agree and believe that shortsighted policies that decrease the incentive for impaired healthcare professionals to enter treatment earlier will only further compromise patient safety. Opponents of these policies argue that since addiction is known to be a chronic, relapsing disease for which there is no cure, allowing healthcare professionals in recovery to continue to practice without requiring them to disclose their recovery statuses presents a significant risk to the public. They note the success rates of programs with close follow-up and monitoring in place and question whether it is ever acceptable to allow healthcare professionals in recovery to practice without these safeguards in place. Supporting such a policy is akin to hoping the problem will go away if we ignore it or make it illegal. We have tried both approaches and neither has worked.

In the summer of 2010, there was continued pressure being applied by lobbying groups representing many state psychiatric associations to encourage the adaptation of legislation that removes the focus on past addiction and substance abuse in favor of addressing the issue of current addiction and abuse. What was in question was the issue of self-incrimination on license applications and renewals.

Since the phrasing of questions designed to elicit information regarding past or current use of illegal drugs is different from state to state, legislation is needed to create a national standard and specifically determine what type of information must be reported in all license applications. In response to this need for policy clarification, individuals in favor of greater regulation point to the many problems with the current policy.

Under the current structure, there is concern that loopholes exist that may allow impaired healthcare professionals to move from one state to another without having to disclose their addiction histories. Proponents of shifting policy toward more regulation point out that after receiving treatment through voluntary admission to an impaired professionals program, there are no records that follow healthcare professionals in recovery when they subsequently apply for licenses in other states. There is no mechanism in place that would alert a licensing board to the need to consider possible monitoring or restrictions on a new applicant. Should a relapse occur, the entire process is repeated in the new state and the healthcare professional can simply move along to the next state.

Should the subsequent application be denied, the board that refuses to issue a license is not obligated to disclose publicly why it declined the application. These events, which are not reported if a healthcare professional remains compliant, do not generate a permanent record, which is the point of both proponents and opponents of the status quo. I suggest that this problem can once again be addressed by the creation of national standards for the treatment of addicted healthcare professionals. If there is only one area in which to practice then there are no other states to move to and the loopholes created by individual states licensing their own professionals are closed.

Those who argue for the creation of a permanent record, much like the national practitioner data bank (the electronic repository that currently collects information on adverse licensure actions, certain actions restricting clinical privileges and professional society membership actions taken against physicians, dentists and other practitioners as well as data on all payments made on behalf of physicians in connection with liability settlements and judgments), often cite the doctrine of informed consent. It is this idea that every competent adult individual has the right to determine what will be done with his or her body that guides the relationship between healthcare professionals and their patients.

In order for individuals to consent to a treatment or procedure, they must understand the risks and benefits inherent with the proposed intervention. Patients must be presented with the results of any tests or diagnostic studies that have been performed and healthcare professionals must help the patients to understand their significance. While it is recognized that the depth of understanding related to these issues is considerably greater for healthcare professionals than it is for most patients, all reasonable options should be presented and all of the facts should be given. It has been well established that healthcare professionals who perform interventions or procedures without properly obtaining informed consent are, in fact, committing battery upon the patients. Proponents of this policy change argue that healthcare professionals' statuses as individuals in recovery is of material concern to patients and must be part of the discussion of informed consent. I strongly disagree.

No reasonable person would choose to have a procedure performed by someone who is under the influence, but this issue is different from that of a healthcare professional in recovery. The right of the patient to informed consent must be balanced with the right of the healthcare professional to protect his or her own personal health information.

William, a lawyer who for several decades has been representing physicians defending their medical licenses related to issues with addiction, told me, "This is a problem, there is no doubt about it, but I look at it from the other side of the coin. When I had surgery last year the first person I wanted to talk to was the anesthesiologist. I asked him if he was in recovery, but not because I didn't want a physician in recovery taking care of me. Quite the opposite. I know how big of a problem this is and I know what kind of safeguards are in place for the physician in recovery who has returned to clinical practice. I'd take the anesthesiologist in recovery over the one I don't know about any day of the week."

While some may argue that a healthcare professional in recovery has the obligation to disclose this fact to his or her patients, most people recognize that this is much the same as asking a physician to report his or her level of competence with a given procedure during the consent process. Although there are some who will rightfully inform patients that they do not have sufficient experience to perform an operation and refer them to colleagues with greater skill, this is not always the case. To share this information voluntarily may be difficult and this has been recognized by lawmakers.

Recent legislation has mandated the reporting of metrics designed to allow the public to make an informed decision regarding which hospital or physician to go to for treatment. All of this information is available online and accessible in various forms. Regarding the issue of a healthcare professional with a chronic disease such as addiction that has the potential to interfere with his or her ability to competently care for his or her patients, many of these issues are currently being addressed in the courts. It has been established that addiction to drugs or alcohol does not necessarily translate into negligence but could be considered negligence if the addiction resulted in a lower standard of care.

There is no indication that the increasing rates of addiction to prescription medications are slowing. These drugs are readily available and counterfeit "medications" are being manufactured to meet the needs of prescription drug addicts all over the world. If this continues at its current pace, prescription drugs will soon overtake marijuana as society's most popular illicit drug. Is it only a matter of time before people are more likely to pop prescription pills than to take a drink of alcohol? It is in this context that the risk for addiction in our population of healthcare professionals continues to increase.

Without dramatic changes to the way we educate our healthcare providers about the nature of addiction in both their patients and themselves, we will continue to see an increase in the number of impaired healthcare professionals. Without changes to the curriculums in medical schools and nursing programs to include an emphasis on the identification and treatment of addicted healthcare professionals, we continue to put the physicians and nurses of the future as well as their patients at risk.

I am hopeful that the next decade will see a significant change in the way all healthcare is delivered. As the population continues to age and fewer working people must shoulder the burden of caring for an increasing number of disabled and elderly, reducing the cost of healthcare delivery becomes even more paramount.

Shifting the emphasis from treatment toward prevention will be of great benefit toward reducing the future costs of providing this care, but we cannot allow this to come at the expense of reduced treatment for addiction and other forms of mental illness. To allow the perception to persist that psychiatric illness is somehow less deserving of treatment than other, perhaps better understood, medical conditions is not acceptable. The dismal reimbursement for these services by health insurance companies over the past forty years has only added to the belief that addiction is somehow less of a "real" condition and has led to limited access to these essential services for those unable to afford the costs of treatment.

If we are to have a healthcare system in which excellent care is provided to all citizens, then making the best treatments accessible to as many patients as possible becomes a national priority. In addition, we must protect the people who provide that care and work to detect and provide the best treatments for addicted healthcare professionals. Being treated by an addicted healthcare professional is never acceptable.

Acknowledgements

While conducting the research to write this book, I had the great pleasure to talk with many people who are dealing with the issue of addicted healthcare professionals on a daily basis. These are the people on the front lines of addiction treatment: the people tasked with training new physicians, nurses, dentists, pharmacists and other healthcare professionals and the people tasked with managing addicted healthcare professionals in both treatment and licensing aspects.

Not surprisingly, given the climate of intolerance that surrounds this taboo topic, some of the people to whom I reached out refused to discuss this matter with me directly or simply returned curt one- or two-line answers to specific questions. Despite the potential for controversy, people on both sides of the issue found the courage to make their cases. These individuals, regardless of their stances on the issues of treatment versus license revocation or return to work versus retraining, were willing to share their personal experiences and opinions and for that I am very grateful.

I also wish to acknowledge the large number of healthcare professionals in recovery who enthusiastically shared the details of their personal stories with me for this project. The response to requests for information was overwhelming.

NOTES

Preface

1. Substance Abuse and Mental Health Services Administration, "Results from the 2005 National Survey of Drug Use and Health: National Findings," Office of Applied Studies, Rockville, MD, 2006, http://www .samhsa.gov/data/nsduh/2k5nsduh/2k5results.pdf.
2. Joan M. Brewster, "Prevalence of alcohol and other drug problems among physicians," *Journal of the American Medical Association* 255 (1986): 1913–20.
3. Bruce H. Alexander et al., "Cause-specific Mortality Risks of Anesthesiologists," *Anesthesiology* 93 (2000): 922–30.

PART I: THE SCOPE OF THE EPIDEMIC

Chapter 1: Harm Caused by Addicted Healthcare Professionals

1. Committee on Quality of Health Care in America and Institute of Medicine, *To Err Is Human: Building a Safer Health System*, ed. Linda T. Kohn, Janet M. Corrigan and Molla S. Donaldson (Washington, DC: National Academy Press, 2000).
2. Christopher P. Landrigan et al., "Temporal Trends in Rates of Patient Harm Resulting from Medical

Care," *New England Journal of Medicine* 363 (2010): 2124–2134.

Chapter 2: A Problem More Common Than You Think

1. Deni Carise et al., "Prescription OxyContin abuse among patients entering addiction treatment," *American Journal of Psychiatry* 164 (2007): 1750–1756.
2. Substance Abuse and Mental Health Services Administration, "Results from the 2005 National Survey."
3. International Narcotics Control Board, "Report of the International Narcotics Control Board for 2006," United Nations, 2007, http://www.incb.org/pdf/e/ar/2006/annual-report-2006-en.pdf.
4. David E. Joranson et al., "Trends in medical use and abuse of opioid analgesics," *Journal of the American Medical Association* 283 (2000): 1710–1714.
5. National Drug Intelligence Center, "National Drug Threat Assessment 2011," United States Department of Justice, August 2011, http://www.justice.gov/ndic/pubs44/44849/44849p.pdf.
6. Substance Abuse and Mental Health Services Administration, "Results from the 2009 National Survey of Drug Use and Health: Summary of National Findings," Rockville, MD: Department of Health and Human Services, 2010, http://www.samhsa.gov/data/NSDUH/2k10NSDUH/2k10Results.htm.
7. National Drug Intelligence Center, "National Drug Threat Assessment 2011."
8. Food and Drug Administration Office of Criminal Investigations, "February 24, 2010: Statement by U.S. Attorney David Gaouette Regarding the Sentencing of Kristen Parker," U.S. Department of Justice, http://www.fda.gov/ICECI/CriminalInvestigations/ucm280213.htm.
9. Donald M. Bell et al., "Controlled drug misuse by certified registered nurse anesthetists," *American*

Association of Nurse Anesthetists Journal 67 (1999): 133–140.

10. United States Department of Health and Human Services, National Institutes of Health, National Institute on Alcohol Abuse and Alcoholism, "Alcohol and Other Drugs," *Alcohol Alert* 76 (July 2008), http://www.niaaa .nih.gov/Publications/AlcoholAlerts/Documents/AA76 .pdf.

11. MR Baldisseri, "Impaired healthcare professional." *Critical Care Medicine* 35 (2007): S106–S116.

PART II: HOW HEALTHCARE PROFESSIONALS BECOME ADDICTED

Chapter 4: The Origins of Addiction

1. Centers for Disease Control and Prevention, "Trends in the Prevalence of Sexual Behaviors: National YRBS: 1991–2009," U.S. Department of Health and Human Services, Centers for Disease Control and Prevention, National Center for Chronic Disease Prevention and Health Promotion, Division of Adolescent and School Health, http://www.cdc.gov/healthyyouth/yrbs/pdf/us _sexual_trend_yrbs.pdf.

Chapter 5: Why Some Healthcare Professionals Become Addicted

1. American Medical Association, "Report of the Board of Trustees," *Journal of the American Medical Association* 162 (1956): 750.

2. Amy R. Mohn, Wei-Dong Yao and Marc G. Caron, "Genetic and genomic approaches to reward and addiction," *Neuropharmacology* 47 (2004): 101–10; Mary Jeanne Kreek, David A. Nielsen and K. Steven LaForge, "Genes associated with addiction: alcoholism, opiate, and

cocaine addiction," *NeuroMolecular Medicine* 5 (2004): 85–108.

3. National Institute on Drug Abuse, "Genetics: the blueprint of health and disease," National Institute on Drug Abuse, April 2008, http://www.drugabuse.gov/publications/topics-in-brief/genetics-addiction.

4. N. Hiroi and S. Agatsuma, "Genetic susceptibility to substance dependence," *Molecular Psychiatry* 10 (2005): 336–44.

5. Dan J. Lettieri, "Drug Abuse: A review of explanations and models of explanation," in *Alcohol and Substance Abuse in Adolescence,* edited by Barry Stimmel (New York: Haworth, 1985): 9–40.

6. Athina Markou, TR Kosten and GF Koob, "Neurobiological similarities in depression and drug dependence: a self-medication hypothesis," *Neuropsychopharmacology* 18 (1998): 135–74; EP Nace, CW Davis and JP Gaspari, "Axis II comorbidity in substance abusers," *American Journal of Psychiatry* 148 (1991): 118–20.

7. Paul E. Wischmeyer et al., "A Survey of Propofol Abuse in Academic Anesthesia Programs," *Anesthesia and Analgesia* 105 (2007): 1066–71.

8. Patrick H. Hughes et al., "Resident physician substance use, by specialty," *American Journal of Psychiatry* 149 (1992): 1348–54.

9. MM Udel, "Chemical abuse/dependence: Physicians' occupational hazard," *Journal of the Medical Association of Georgia* 73 (1984): 775–8.

10. Mark S. Gold, Joanne A. Byars and Kimberly Frost-Pineda, "Occupational exposure and addictions for physicians: case studies and theoretical implications," *Psychiatric Clinics North America* 27 (2004): 745–53.

11. Mark S. Gold et al., "Fentanyl abuse and dependence: further evidence for second hand exposure hypothesis," *Journal of Addictive Diseases* 25 (2006): 15–21.

Chapter 6: What Types of Prescription Drugs Healthcare Professionals Abuse

1. Office of Applied Studies, Substance Abuse and Mental Health Services Administration, "Heroin—Changes in how it is used: 1995–2005," *The DASIS Report,* April 26, 2007, http://www.samhsa.gov/data/2k7/heroinTX/heroinTX.pdf.

2. Ilkka Ojanpera et al., "Blood levels of 3-methylfentanyl in 3 fatal poisoning cases," *American Journal of Forensic Medicine and Pathology,* 27(2006): 328–331.

3. Ethan O. Bryson and Jeffrey H. Silverstein, "Addiction and substance abuse in anesthesiology," *Anesthesiology* 109 (2008): 905–17.

4. Joranson et al., "Trends in medical use and abuse of opioid analgesics."

5. Aaron M. Gilson et al., "A reassessment of trends in the medical use and abuse of opioid analgesics and implications for diversion control: 1997–2002," *Journal of Pain and Symptom Management* 28 (2004): 176–188.

6. SAMHSA, "Prescription Drug Abuse Rises: SAMHSA and FDA Educate Public," *SAMHSA News* 11 (2003).

7. Centers for Disease Control and Prevention, "Emergency department visits involving nonmedical use of selected prescription drugs—United States, 2004–2008," *Morbidity and Mortality Weekly Report* 59 (2010): 705–709.

8. James D. Colliver et al., "Misuse of Prescription Drugs: Data From the 2002, 2003, and 2004 National Surveys on Drug Use and Health," DHHS Publication No. SMA 06–4192, Analytic Series A–28, Rockville, Maryland: SAMHSA, Office of Applied Studies, 2006.

9. Substance Abuse and Mental Health Services Administration, "Results from the 2008 National Survey on Drug Use and Health: National Findings," Office of Applied Studies, NSDUH Series H–36, HHS Publication

No. SMA 09–4434, Rockville, MD, 2009, http://www
.oas.samhsa.gov/nsduh/2k8nsduh/2k8Results.pdf.

PART III: PROTECTING YOURSELF FROM ADDICTED HEALTHCARE PROFESSIONALS

Chapter 7: Identifying Addicted Healthcare Professionals

1. Richard H. Epstein, David M. Gratch and Zvi Grunwald, "Development of a scheduled drug diversion surveillance system based on an analysis of atypical drug transactions," *Anesthesia and Analgesia* 105 (2007): 1053–60.
2. G. Douglas Talbott, "The impaired physician and intervention: A key to recovery," *Journal of the Florida Medical Association* 69 (1992): 793–7.

Chapter 8: Reporting Impaired Healthcare Professionals

1. *Kadlec Medical Center vs Lakeview Anesthesia Associates*, 527 F.3d 412 (5th Cir. 2008).
2. *Lakeview Anesthesia Associates, et al., Petitioners v. Kadlec Medical Center, et al.* No. 08-375, United States Supreme Court December 1, 2008.

Chapter 9: Legal Issues and Addicted Healthcare Professionals

1. AMA Council on Mental Health, "The Sick Physician: impairment by psychiatric disorders, including alcoholism and drug dependence," *Journal of the American Medical Association* 223 (1973): 684–687.
2. Oregon State Medical Board, "HPP—Health Professionals Program: History and Background," Oregon.gov, www.oregon.gov/OMB/healthprog.shtml (accessed 02/25/2012).

3. Heather Hamza and Ethan O. Bryson, "Buprenorphine maintenance therapy in the opioid addicted Healthcare Professional returning to clinical practice—a hidden controversy," Mayo Clinic Proceedings, March 2012.

4. *Americans with Disabilities Act of 1990*, Pub. L. No. 101-336, § 2, 104 Stat. 328 (1991).

5. Laurence M. Westreich, "Addiction and the Americans with Disabilities Act," *Journal of the American Academy of Psychiatry and the Law* 30 (2002): 355–63.

6. Jeffrey L. Metzner and James B. Buck, "Psychiatric disability determinations and personal injury litigation," in *Principles and Practice of Forensic Psychiatry*, edited by Richard Rosner (London: Arnold, 2003): 672–84.

PART IV: HELP AND RECOVERY FOR ADDICTED HEALTHCARE PROFESSIONALS

Chapter 10: Treatment Programs for Healthcare Professionals

1. Phyllis A. Harrison and Stephen E. Asche, "Comparison of substance abuse treatment outcomes for inpatients and outpatients," *Journal of Substance Abuse Treatment* 17 (October 1999): 207–20; Marion Malivert et al., "Effectiveness of therapeutic communities: a systematic review," *European Addiction Research* 18 (2012): 1–11; SC Oudejans et al., "Five years of ROM in substance abuse treatment centres in the Netherlands," *Tijdschrift voor psychiatrie* 54 (2012): 185–90; Gregory E Skipper, Michael D. Campbell and Robert L. DuPont, "Anesthesiologists with Substance Use Disorders: A 5-Year Outcome Study from 16 State Physician Health Programs," *Anesthesia and Analgesia* 109 (2009): 891–896.

2. A. Thomas McLellan et al., "Five year outcomes in a cohort study of physicians treated for substance use disorders in the United States," *British Medical Journal*

337 (November 2008): a2038; Robert L. DuPont et al., "Setting the standard for recovery: Physicians' Health Programs," *Journal of Substance Abuse Treatment* 36 (March 2009): 159–71.

3. Robert L. DuPont et al., "How are addicted physicians treated? A national survey of Physician Health Programs," *Journal of Substance Abuse Treatment* 37 (July 2009): 1–7.

4. Paul Guerino, Paige M. Harrison and William J. Sabol, "Prisoners in 2010," *National Criminal Justice* 236096 (December 2011) http://bjs.ojp.usdoj.gov/content/pub/pdf/p10.pdf.

Chapter 11: Alternative Professional Health Programs

1. AMA Council on Mental Health, "The Sick Physician."

2. G. Douglas Talbott et al., "The Medical Association of Georgia's Impaired Physicians Program Review of the first 1,000 Physicians: Analysis of Specialty," *Journal of the American Medical Association* 257 (1987): 2927–30.

3. Hamza and Bryson, "Buprenorphine maintenance therapy."

4. P. Kintz et al., "Evidence of addiction by anesthesiologists as documented by hair analysis," *Forensic Science International* 153 (2005): 81–4.

5. American Nurses Association, "The Profession's Response to the Problem of Addictions and Psychiatric Disorders in Nursing," American Nurses Association, 2002, http://nursingworld.org/MainMenuCategories/WorkplaceSafety/Work-Environment/ImpairedNurse/Response.pdf (accessed 02/25/2012).

6. T. Monroe, F. Pearson and H. Kenaga, "Procedures for handling cases of substance abuse among nurses: A comparison of disciplinary and alternative programs," *Journal of Addictions Nursing* 19 (2008): 156–161.

7. Ibid.

Chapter 12: Recovery and Prospects for Returning to Work

1. John V. Booth et al., "Substance abuse among physicians: a survey of academic anesthesiology programs," *Anesthesia and Analgesia* 95 (2002): 1024–30.
2. Ethan O. Bryson, "Should anesthesia residents with a history of substance abuse be allowed to continue training in clinical anesthesia? The results of a survey of anesthesia residency program directors," *Journal of Clinical Anesthesia* 21 (2009): 508–13.
3. Gregory B. Collins et al., "Chemical dependency treatment outcomes of residents in anesthesiology: results of a survey," *Anesthesia and Analgesia* 101 (2005): 1457–62.
4. Karen B. Domino et al., "Risk factors for relapse in healthcare professionals with substance use disorders," *Journal of the American Medical Association* 293 (2005): 1453–60.
5. Ethan O. Bryson and Heather Hamza, "The drug seeking anesthesia provider," *International Anesthesiology Clinics* 49 (2011): 157–171.
6. McLellan et al., "Five year outcomes in a cohort study of physicians."

PART V: WHAT NEEDS TO BE DONE

Chapter 13: Proactive Measures to Prevent Harm

1. Bryson and Hamza, "The drug seeking anesthesia provider."
2. ASA Task Force on Chemical Dependence of the ASA Committee on Occupational Health of Operating Room Personnel, "Chemical Dependence in Anesthesiologists: What you need to know when you need to know it," 1998, http://anestit.unipa.it/mirror/asa2/ProfInfo/chemical.html.

Conclusion: The Need For National Standards And Consistent Policy

1. McLellan et al., "Five year outcomes in a cohort study of physicians"; DuPont et al., "Setting the standard for recovery."